T0093672

Breaking
the Silence

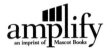

www.amplifypublishing.com

Breaking the Silence: Why Openness About Your Sex Life is the Best Medicine for Your Health, Relationships, and Overall Happiness

This book is not intended as a substitute for the medical advice of physicians. The reader should regularly consult a physician in matters relating to his/her health and particularly with respect to any symptoms that may require diagnosis or medical attention.

The views and opinions expressed in this book are solely those of the author. These views and opinions do not necessarily represent those of the publisher or staff.

Some names and identifying details have been changed to protect the privacy of individuals.

For more information, please contact:
Amplify Publishing
620 Herndon Parkway #320
Herndon, VA 20170
info@amplifypublishing.com

Library of Congress Control Number: 2020909661

CPSIA Code: PRFRE1020A
ISBN-13: 978-1-64543-467-2

Printed in Canada

*To my loving wife, who has given me
everything a man could ever dream to have.*

Breaking
the
Silence

Why Openness About Your Sex Life
is the Best Medicine for Your Health,
Relationships, and Overall Happiness

Moshe Kedan, MD

CONTENTS

INTRODUCTION

I t was my first meeting with a new patient—a woman who came in for a routine physical examination. Women are more interested in their health than men are and more willing to try preventive measures to stay healthy, and they usually make more of an effort and pay better attention to their bodies. This woman was fifty years old and a mother of three, and she told me that she had been happily married for twenty-six years to her husband, who was fifty-two and the chief executive of a reputable company.

I usually start with a medical interview to learn the pertinent health information that can assist me in helping the patient. Then I progress to the "review of systems" that every physician learns how to do in medical school. I asked this patient about her digestion, vision, hearing, breathing, bathroom habits, exercise, diet—taking a complete history of every system of her body. However, I didn't stop, like other physicians usually do, at her sexual system. When I asked this woman about her sex life, she openly responded that the frequency of sexual activity by her and her husband had decreased to once or twice a month.

When I inquired why, she said, "I have less interest in sex, and my priority is to take care of my children." When I asked about her husband, she said, "He is a good father and a good husband, and I love him very much." Then, when I asked about the low frequency of their sexual encounters, she said, "Of course, he would like to have it more often, but he *understands*." When I asked what she meant by "he understands," she could not answer. It was obvious to me that, really, she was hoping her husband understood, when in fact, it was *she* who did not understand *him*.

I cannot tell you how many times I have heard some variation on this, most often from women but also from men. Sex has become infrequent, they're not happy, but they really love their partner. Nevertheless, the problems persist and only get bigger with time. What does this have to do with the bigger picture of health? I will get to that.

At this stage of the conversation, I moved to my physical examination. The woman proved to be healthy, and after she was dressed, we spoke more about her sex life. I learned that she was not happy to have gained ten pounds and that she was feeling fatigued and not motivated to exercise. She said that her husband seemed to be more short-tempered and anxious with her, but she attributed this to the stress of his job.

After talking about the other results of my examination, I asked whether she and her husband had ever discussed their feelings about their sex lives. Her response was one I've become very familiar with: "We don't talk about sex, but we love each other and care for each other. I have less interest in sex than he does, and he wants more, but he understands." I knew that most likely her husband did not "understand," and that this misreading of her spouse was probably having a negative impact on her marriage.

I asked, "What is he supposed to do when his sexual desire is active and he wants to find comfort through lovemaking with you?" I explained that men's sexuality can remain strong throughout their lives, that it is normal for a man her husband's age to have a strong sexual desire, and that it is important that it be satisfied. It is also a sign of good health. Then I said, "But if that desire is not naturally fulfilled, it will affect his happiness and may turn into frustration that negatively affects his attitude and behavior toward you and your marriage." I told her that wanting frequent sex doesn't make a man unusual; it makes him normal.

The patient was looking uncomfortable, and I said, "When you say that he understands, do you mean that he should suppress his sexual passion toward you or be with other women?" It was obvious that this woman had never had this kind of conversation with anyone—especially her doctor—had never confronted the situation, and hadn't taken the time to think about what was going on in her husband's mind and heart. However, she didn't become angry with me about my questions. She clearly welcomed them.

She suddenly broke into tears. I waited until she gathered her emotions, and then she said, "I am so sorry; I love my husband. He is my life, and I care for him, and I feel so bad that I've let him down." We spoke some more about the importance of sexual relations in a relationship, and at the conclusion of our visit, she hugged me and thanked me for caring enough to ask those questions. She promised that she would try to talk with her husband and get them to open up to each other about their intimate life.

A RARE AND NEEDED CONVERSATION

FOR MOST PRIMARY CARE PHYSICIANS, this would have been an unusual conversation. But for me, it has become a commonplace one. I have been practicing medicine for forty-five years, and it has become clear to me that many of the mental and physical problems that people experience—the things that bring them into my office in the first place—are either caused or exacerbated by the stress, frustrations, and emotional suffering that come with sexual dysfunction within a relationship. Sex remains something that couples don't talk about, even in the privacy of their beds. The secrecy, shame, and hostility that often build up when sex is poor, infrequent, neglected, or disregarded can damage people's health, destroy their marriages, and ruin their lives. I have seen it happen, and it is unnecessary.

Here's another example. A man, age forty-eight, came to see me for high blood pressure, something I treat frequently. But as part of our conversation about his well-being, I asked the same questions about his marriage and his intimate life. Why do I do this? One good reason is that sexual problems are sometimes the main factor behind physical or functional disorders. But I have also become convinced that my patients' well-being depends not only on treating them for their medical conditions but also on helping them find the path to happiness, and one of the keys to happiness is a healthy, satisfying sex life.

It turned out that this man was worried that his wife, aged forty-four, might have an affair. His marriage wasn't happy, and after some more careful conversation, he finally admitted, defensively, that he was having trouble maintaining an erection.

As it is for many men, this perceived failure had been devastating for him. It had thrown him into a downward spiral of embarrassment, worry, defeat, guilt, and emasculation. As often happens, his anxiety over his performance led to recurring erectile dysfunction (ED) as fear took its own course and kept building. There was nothing wrong with him physically, but his fear became a self-fulfilling prophecy. By the time I saw him, he was worried that his wife would leave because he couldn't satisfy her sexually. But he had never spoken about the problem with anyone—including his wife—because of his shame.

Instead, he tried to avoid sexual encounters, using all sorts of excuses to conceal his fear of embarrassment. It is understandable. Imagine any man, together in bed with his loving wife, both ready to enjoy sexual intimacy, and at the peak of arousal, he becomes unable to perform. Efforts to "make it work" end in failure. Now this poor man is lying in the dark, paralyzed with humiliation, with no help. He feels nothing but shame, embarrassment, and guilt, though he has done nothing wrong. His wife, unaware of how devastating this is for him, has no idea how to support him. His only option is to escape and avoid more intimate encounters.

This silence, this taboo over the topic of sexuality, sexual performance, loss of sex drive . . . it is an epidemic. These are just two cases of thousands that I have encountered in my years in medicine, and while all have their unique features, they share one unfortunate thing in common: *No physician had ever asked these men or women about their sex lives before I did.*

Asking a few simple questions about their sexuality opened a door surrounded by secrecy, mystery, and shame for these men and women. By inviting people to talk about their intimate lives in such a simple way, I discovered the truth about their feelings, happiness, and fears that I could not have ever discovered using the routine questionnaires that all physicians have patients complete upon their arrival at the office. I saw and learned how people handled their sexual issues, in good ways and bad ways, and the consequences. What I've learned has led me to write this book to share this information for the benefit of all.

In medical school we learn about the human body as a collection of systems—cardiovascular, immune, digestive, endocrine, musculoskeletal, nervous, and so on. But the human body is incredibly complex, and in order to make it possible for medical students to learn an already overwhelming amount of information, instructors tell them, "This assembly of systems is all the patient is," as though a human being can be reduced to interconnected machinery like an automobile. In the medical field, we have the tendency to deal with what we know and learn from books while trying to ignore the parts that we don't know. This can make us feel powerful, but unfortunately, it also gives the false impression that physicians should know it all. If something goes wrong, it must be the physician's error.

But with all our progress, which has helped cure disease and prolong life, we know perhaps 5 percent of what is really going on in our complex bodies. Dealing solely with what we know may make physicians feel comfortable, but it means that we can disregard the power that exists inside our bodies, which has the capability to both heal us or, if ignored or wrongly used, to destroy our health and happiness.

In doing this, medicine ignores the *whole person* behind the patient, the human being with emotions, fears, hopes, and a mind that can and does influence his or her health in many ways. It dismisses important forces like love and sex as powerful factors not only in physical wellness but in overall well-being. That approach does a disservice to both patients and physicians. It reduces the benefits of modern medicine to patients because they end up coming to a doctor's office for the equivalent of an oil change—check their blood pressure, cholesterol, and blood sugar and put some air in the tires—and leave with the same anxiety, stress, and depression that they arrived with.

Patients expect and deserve the physician's time and full attention during their visit. However, this is not available to most patients and therefore creates a crisis in the delivery of medical care. If you ask people how happy they are with the current system of medical care, most will attest that they are not happy about either the time their physician spends with them or the difficult communication with the physician's office. Moreover, the costs of health insurance, deductibles, and drugs have all escalated.

This situation reduces physicians to technicians for whom healing means prescribing a pill, another blood test, and another scan—and who spend much of their time producing electronic medical records for insurance companies in order to be paid and additionally to be protected in the event of a lawsuit for malpractice. The majority of physicians really wish to help their patients but end up with frustrating conflicts between their wishes and the legal, financial, and clerical demands of simply running a practice.

TALKING AND LISTENING ARE THE KEYS

I BEGAN ASKING ABOUT MY patients' sex lives early in my medical career because I realized that the extent of the information I did not know about human well-being was far greater than what I did know. What I found about human sexuality surprised me: not only were patients not offended that I asked about their sexuality, they were delighted that someone was finally asking them about it and integrating the information into the overall picture of their wellness.

One of my most interesting findings is that while women might be intelligent, educated, and devoted to their husbands and marriages, they can do great harm because they have never been educated or guided in understanding their sexual physiology and its connection to their mental and physical well-being. The main factor that all women encounter through life is their libido (sexual desire). This topic is still not well understood in medical science and therefore rarely discussed. The woman is left alone with her changing libido, so she has no chance of understanding it or handling its effect on her health and relationships. She may bring her concerns to her ob-gyn and get hormonal cream or pills, but basically, she will be left to her instincts in how to handle issues like the loss of sexual desire and how that affects her happiness. Changes in libido in women are universal, and will be experienced by every woman throughout her life.

Consequently, when women encounter these changes in their libido with little comprehension about what is happening and why with no guidance on how to respond, the encounter often leads them down a negative path. They can experience depression, loss of self-esteem, motivation, and feminine identity, and feel unattractive sexually, causing them to withdraw from sexual activities.

Sex for a woman is not just orgasm; it is also a powerful driver of her self-confidence and positive behavior, but most importantly, of being in control of her body and her life. When it becomes a negative force, it can be detrimental to her marital life and family union. Her instinct will compel her to reduce or abate her sexual response to her partner, unintentionally overlooking the sexual interests and needs of her husband. As I have seen many, many times in my practice, this response, although not intended, can over time endanger her marriage.

Women need to understand that their libido will change and may diminish over time, even though some women may often feel desire into advanced age. Instead of surrendering to this reality, they can explore the reasons for it, talk with their husbands about what it means to have a healthy sex life, and in some cases, actually regain their previous interest in sex. Libido may decrease beyond normal age and hormonal changes due to stress, poor sleep, medication, and poor marital relations. Similarly, it may increase due to exercise, better marital relations, or changes in diet and daily routine. This means that, despite the fact that the medical profession has no clear understanding of the female libido, it can be treated.

Men have their own sexual issues. Men live in terror of ED, a condition which is often mistakenly viewed as a "disease" against the backdrop of widespread advertising for revenue-generating prescription medications over the past two decades.[1] Men go through an enormous emotional crisis surrounding their sexual performance—which, for many men, defines their masculinity—but its causes and effects are not discussed, so men become fearful that they will lose their capacity and their loving partner, and become sexually handicapped. Commercials, doctors' offices, ED products—the entire topic is treated with secrecy, which tells men that the inability to get an erection is something to be ashamed of. Either that, or it's a subject to joke about.

It is neither. According to the Cleveland Clinic, about 52 percent of American men experience ED, with about 40 percent of men at age forty having occasional episodes of what used to be called "impotence."[2] Call it what you like, but it remains common. It can be due to physical changes or psychological problems, but what ED is not is a sign that a man is less than a man. But men don't believe this because in our daily life, ED is attached to the stigma not just of incapacity but of being less than a man, which causes men to suffer emotionally.

The first sexual "failure" can occur for a man of any age at any time, and it may be meaningless, related to fatigue, anxiety, conflict with a partner, and other factors. However, it may be perceived by a man as an alarm signal that he has a real problem. That will open the door for panic, fear, and concern. The cycle may develop momentum and create the false monster of impotence that leads to a cascade of worries: the response of his spouse, a loss of self-confidence and ambition, the effect on his relationship, and more. I have counseled so many men who were completely broken emotionally by ED and driven in a negative life direction that affected their marriages, careers, and health.

None of this is necessary. So much can change if people simply talk openly about their sexuality and their concerns and if physicians are willing to ask the right questions and listen. But before I go too far into that, here is some background information.

A COMPLEX, DELICATE COLLABORATION

SEXUAL FUNCTION DEPENDS ON THREE physiological systems working together in collaboration. First, the endocrine system produces hormones like testosterone or estrogen that respond to arousing stimuli, which could be anything from a fragrance to suggestive language. The circulatory system dilates in response to hormonal signals and sends blood to the sexual organs, causing them to become engorged and aroused. The nervous system, which detects arousal, sends signals of arousal and pleasure between the brain and the genitals and other sensitive areas of the body (the nipple, the lips, and so on) to get this complex process going.

This three-system process is one of the most delicate and complex in the body and can be thrown off by a wide range of distractions, from embarrassment to postmenopausal hormonal changes to alcohol consumption to children interrupting in the middle of foreplay to some medications. Sexuality is as much a psychological process as a physical one. It flows through three distinct stages.

1. **Libido.** The libido, or sex drive, is where things begin. It's the person's desire for sexual activity. When you wake up in the middle of the night and suddenly want to have sex with your partner, that's your libido talking.

2. **Arousal.** The three systems I mentioned earlier work together to get you aroused. The skin flushes, the pupils dilate, the penis becomes erect, the nipples and the vaginal tissue become engorged, and having sex *now* becomes imperative.

3. **Climax.** One or both partners achieve physical satisfaction and sexual release, often involving orgasm. Orgasm is the most important part of sex for men, but according to a study published in 2017, only about 18 percent of women were able to reach orgasm through intercourse alone,[3] while between 10 and 40 percent of women say they have trouble reaching orgasm even with additional stimulation.[4]

However, this process is delicate and fragile, and a host of emotional and personal factors can disrupt it and ruin the couple's sexual experience. For instance, let's go back to the male patient I talked about before. I tested his physical systems and found them all normal. He wasn't taking medication that caused his sexual dysfunction, either. His impotence had to be psychological.

I reassured him that there was nothing wrong with him, pre-scribed Viagra to help him get past the mental block, and told him, "You are going to function, as I see no medical reason causing the problem." I use Viagra to help men get past the anxiety that can cause impotence, but it was the trust that I built up with him that made him believe my reassurance and respond. Through that trust, improvement became possible. Six months later, he came back to see me. Sex was better. His marriage was better. He said, "I rarely use the Viagra now, to tell you the truth, Doctor. I think I can do without it." The marriage was saved, his fear dissipated, and he regained his confidence.

It really was that simple. Sexual dysfunction in one partner affects the other partner, and eventually both can experience emotional and physical impairment. Often, when sex improves, intimacy and bonding improve. Communication gets better, and stress, anger, and depression disappear.

RESOLVING SEXUAL PROBLEMS IMPROVES HEALTH

I HAVE WRITTEN THIS BOOK because physicians are missing a major factor for health and happiness: a healthy sex life for men and women. In my career I have seen hundreds of families broken apart because no one talked about their sexual needs or dysfunction until it was too late. I don't want to see divorce and pain caused by what is, at its core, a communication problem caused by no one being willing to take the first step.

How do I know this is a problem, apart from what I have seen in four decades of practice? Well, consider that in one large international study including twenty-seven thousand men and women, more than half had experienced some kind of sexual problem, but only 19 percent had talked to a doctor and only 9 percent had been asked by their doctor about their sexual health over a three-year period.[5] That's outrageous. Furthermore, in medical practice there is no clear direction on who to talk to about sexual problems, so patients believe that they should talk to specialists like urologists and gynecologists. But the first line of defense should be a sympathetic primary care doctor who initiates the process as part of the overall exam and health review and recommends a specialist if needed. Urologists and gynecologists are geared to deal with diseases or disorders related to their field, not to sympathetically analyze the lifestyle and emotions of their patients.

Why the primary care physician (PCP)? Because sexual dysfunction can be a sign of more serious underlying conditions, including diabetes, cardiovascular disease, hypertension, hormonal imbalances, prostate disorders, clinical depression, or the beginning of menopause.[6] Any of those conditions can lead to low libido, inability to perform, and other sexual problems in men or women. If you are experiencing sexual dysfunction, it's important to see your physician to make sure it's not a sign of some greater underlying problem.

However, few doctors talk about the reverse of this situation: health problems that can result from sexual dysfunction. In my years of practice, I have had many patients come to me with conditions such as hypertension, depression, anxiety, headaches, insomnia, irritable bowel syndrome, panic attacks, heart palpitations, and other physical symptoms closely linked to psychological and emotional stress. Many enjoyed *complete* relief from their symptoms—yes, complete relief—after simply opening up to me about the sexual problems they were experiencing in their relationships, finding out there was hope, communicating with their partners, and taking the small steps I recommended, which included such things as taking Viagra temporarily, exercising and losing weight together, or changing certain medications.

That should tell you the power sexuality has over our happiness. Many of the common health problems people experience can be traced back to the anxiety, stress, shame, and anger that accompany sexual dysfunction. Men and women suffer terribly when they feel like they are failing their partner or not getting the sexual satisfaction they need, and they often suffer in silence and isolation. The difference that comes when they talk about it with me and with each other and then take action is life changing. Marriages are saved. Lives are saved. Happiness is back, knocking at their door.

PEOPLE NEED TO TALK; DOCTORS NEED TO ASK

DESPITE THESE POSITIVE RESULTS, I have found that few people feel comfortable initiating a conversation with their primary care physician about their ability to get an erection or their lack of sexual desire. Why? Largely, it is because medical culture does not encourage physicians to ask about sexuality, so the discussion has become taboo between doctor and patient—something that remains unspoken by mutual assumption, even though patients might discuss details that are just as sensitive with their physician, such as bowel habits, depression, or conceiving a child. Therefore, in the event that patients encounter sexual problems or questions, they are left alone with their struggle.

The reality is that it is natural and expected for all of us to encounter difficulties, questions, or functional obstacles that should be addressed to an experienced person or professional who can help, guide, educate, or search for a solution. Sexuality is one of those areas, and there is no reason why patients should feel shame or embarrassment when talking about sexual difficulties or questions with their doctors. I have also found that when I have initiated the conversation, patients were not only willing to talk but eager to discuss sexuality.

Physicians are also part of this problem, both in how we are taught and how many of us are forced to run our practices. The average PCP has about fifteen minutes to spend with each patient, and the PCP has to spend that time inputting basic health information into an electronic device. That's how the physician gets paid. But this "assembly line" approach to medicine discourages intimate discussions about sensitive subjects like sex. Also, because of our training, too many physicians treat patients as a set of symptoms instead of respecting and evaluating the whole person and working to heal that person in body and mind. I regularly see patients who tell me they have seen several different physicians, like eye doctors, orthopedists, and dermatologists. Each physician examines a different system, but no one is looking at them as a *person*.

Yes, we are built physiologically of many systems and trillions of cells that work together in serving our life. However, every system is connected to the others and affects the others. Beyond that, every cell in our body speaks with billions of other cells in any given moment. The example I give to demonstrate this is simple. If I take a pin and jab you in the toe, your whole body will get the message: you will retract your leg without thinking about it, your face will express discomfort, and you may scream. Every cell in our body is interconnected. Therefore, as physicians, we cannot omit one system in our body and treat it like it is isolated, intimate, and personal.

This type of thinking leaves the patient alone to struggle with his "personal-intimate" problem. For us as physicians, by excluding the sexual system from our patient examination, we are leaving a hole in care that unfortunately could be very important to our ability to understand the patient and remedy his or her problem.

Therefore, I decided forty-five years ago to break this taboo and include the sexual system in my inquiry and make the review of this system an integral part of my examination. I have carried that through my practice as physician, and I am finally ready to share my experience and my findings for the benefit of both physicians and patients.

Can't people go see sex therapists? Certainly, and they may help resolve some psychological issues. However, sex therapists can't help with the physiological and medical factors because they lack the training and the medical background. What's more, they can be hard to find and are usually expensive and not covered by insurance. They can take care of people who already know that they have specific sexual problems, but only a physician can discover the problems in those who are not aware of their problems when they visit the doctor for something else.

Long ago, when I opened my practice in Clearwater, Florida, I determined that I would do things differently. First of all, I resolved to remain humble in the face of all that I do not know about the human body and human health—many things, as the medical profession has very limited knowledge. As a result, I treat the patient not as a collection of systems and symptoms but as a whole person. To quote the Hebrew Talmud, "I have learned from my colleagues more than I learned from my teachers, but from my students I have learned the most." To me, that means that I have learned more in medicine from my patients than I ever did in medical school, reading research, or consulting with my colleagues.

I respect my patients, as they are my real teachers. They show me what they feel, what they think, and what works the best, or what does not work for their problems. That is also how modern medicine has evolved: observation of large numbers of patients and learning from their responses to new treatments.

I've learned by spending time with my patients face to face, asking lots of questions, and listening. On average I spend forty-five minutes with new patients, asking them about their systems, their lives, their sleep, their marriages, and their sexuality. That builds up the most valuable part of the doctor-patient relationship and the most powerful healing tool I have: *trust*. When that trust exists between me and the patients, it creates a healing power, an important tool to use in helping each patient. They relax with me and share their feelings so they can describe their pain and their problems. They accept my help, trust it, and use it as a tool to achieve comfort in a moment of fear and uncertainty. They allow me to offer them a new perspective on situations they may have dealt with for years.

With all those intimate conversations and trust, these are the patterns I have come to recognize:

- Couples misunderstand sex, arousal, desire, and orgasm. They are left in the dark about desire and arousal change over the years, and they are ignorant of the role that sex plays in a healthy relationship. Because of this, the inevitable sexual changes that come with time lead to blame, guilt, paranoia, fear, anxiety, and resentment that create health problems and destroy marriages.

- Many couples believe that if they experience problems with sex, there is nothing that can be done. They have to live with it. But that's not true.

- Too few couples speak candidly with each other about their own sexual needs or problems, the amount of sex they desire (or don't desire), what turns them on in bed, and other matters that seem normal subjects for discussion between people who share a bed and share life together.

- Most physicians don't offer much help because they aren't trained in sexuality and don't know the right questions to ask. They aren't paid by the health care system for the extra time it takes to explore this area and are often embarrassed by the subject.

- Sex is still a taboo subject in general. Think about how sex is used to smear competitors, especially in politics. It has also become associated with the harassment and abuse of women. No wonder most physicians want to stay far away from this topic!

- Physicians are not gaining confidence or experience with their patients in the area of sexuality because they are excluding sexuality from their routine encounters with patients. This reluctance makes patients hesitant, creating a cycle of shame and concealment. Women are much more open to discussing their sexuality, while men are more reserved and closed. It often takes a longer time to get clear information from men, which can hinder care.

But I believe the solution is clear. First, we must open our eyes to the role that sexual health plays in overall well-being and to the ways that our sexuality changes over time. Next, we must challenge the myths and taboos about male and female sexuality and make it easier to talk openly about the changes and challenges each person faces. We must encourage each other to speak openly and honestly about our sexual needs and desires without shame or guilt. Finally, we need to teach primary care physicians to speak candidly to their patients about their sex lives and to treat human sexuality as an important part of overall wellness—another important physiological system that has just as much impact on overall well-being as the nervous system or the cardiovascular system.

WHAT I HOPE TO ACCOMPLISH WITH THIS BOOK

FIRST, I WANT TO let you know everything that I have learned from ordinary patients coming to me for various medical issues. None of these patients ever came to me to ask about or be treated for sexual problems. The information that I obtained from them was always in response to my inquiry about their sexuality. Surprisingly to many of my colleagues (but not to me), all my patients were open to my inquiry, volunteered to answer, and were eager to participate, and most were appreciative and happy to follow my method of thinking.

I want to highlight the emotional and relationship agony that men and women feel when they experience sexual dysfunction; to make the world aware of the ways that dysfunction negatively affects their marriages, careers, lifestyles, and physical health; and to let people know that those problems can be addressed. I also want to paint a clear picture of the value of a patient-centric approach to practicing medicine—an approach built around physicians spending more time talking with their patients about anything they express, gaining their trust and discussing their intimate lives—and I want to show how eager most people are to talk to someone objective about their sexual problems.

I wish to share what some of these wonderful men and women said to me with such sincerity and anguish—share why they said it and what it meant—and share how I addressed them and the advice I gave them.

I also aspire to show readers how health is linked to sexuality and how health problems are so often linked to the secrecy and despair that commonly accompany troubles with performance or libido. I wish to enlighten my fellow physicians about the ways they can transform their own practices, not to mention their experience in medicine and their patient outcomes, by giving respect to these very real sexual issues.

Most of all, I want to let couples at every age and every stage of life know that no matter how embarrassing or intractable their problems with sex might seem, no matter how much they fight or how much they have given up—there is *hope*. There are always things they can do. They do not need to watch their marriage disintegrate; resign themselves to a future without sex; adopt negative habits like smoking, gambling, or drinking; or cheat on each other. There is much that can be done to encourage communication, break the taboos, and see real change.

I want to save marriages and improve lives by helping couples understand the vital role sex plays in well-being and in the strength of the family union. I want to help people connect their sexuality with their health, satisfaction, and happiness. I want to help doctors see patients as whole people and educate them on the vital role they have to play. I want everyone to see sex as a God-given gift—or, as the Bible says, "I gave you the good and the bad, and you chose the good."

In the Song of Solomon (6:3), scripture reads, "I am my beloved's and my beloved is mine." That is the simple meaning of love and pure human sexuality.

I want to heal people. That is what physicians do.

Thank you for joining me. Let's begin.

Chapter One

WHY DON'T WE TALK ABOUT SEX?

Perhaps one of the reasons we are so reluctant to talk about sex is that we are having less of it. A landmark 2017 study[1] led by Jean Twenge, a psychology professor at San Diego State University, found that Americans are having less sex than we did from 1995 to 1999. Distressingly, the biggest drops in sexual activity are among married couples (twice as high as in single people) and in people between the ages of fifty and fifty-nine—exactly the age group that comes to me most often complaining that they are no longer having satisfying sex. Kate Julian, writing in *The Atlantic,* called the situation a "sex recession."[2]

Nobody is really sure why this is happening. The researchers said that fatigue might be an issue, as men and women are working harder to take care of children while maintaining two careers. Some speculated that people's obsession with their new technology, including multiple choices of television programs, smart phones, and other devices, could be part of the problem, and that seems more likely to me. If you're a man worried about ED or a woman who fears asking her husband why he has no interest in sex, being on your iPhone gives you a built-in way to avoid interaction. This results in the opposite of the intimate communication that's necessary to sustain a marriage. Sex is an interdependent process; it requires both the man and woman to be open to each other, and if their fear keeps them from communicating about intimacy, sex will not happen.

I am not a sociologist, so I am not going to explore the cultural, social, and psychological factors—from marrying later in life to pornography—that may be causing this alarming trend. What concerns me is that no one is talking about the lack of sex as a public health issue, which it is.

Why has sex become a problem, instead of the rich, wonderful part of life that it should be? I think some of it is due to our culture. Modern life has isolated us from each other. When I first came to the United States in my twenties, interaction was mostly face to face. People talked on front porches, spent time with friends, and watched television sparingly (there were only a few channels available). Today, we live on the Internet and barely leave our homes. Communication online has replaced conversation, and human emotions have been replaced by video clips.

As a result, we've lost our ability to communicate deeply and intimately with each other. We are passing all this to the new generation by providing them with smart phones and video games early in life. They're losing their ability to read faces and understand unspoken expression. That's damaged the family unit, with 40 to 50 percent of first marriages ending up in divorce, according to the American Psychological Association.[3] Families often come to an end with two lawyers in court and brokenhearted, traumatized children. And since about 60 percent of families have both the man and woman working,[4] sex becomes an afterthought. Husband and wife are too exhausted and stressed to care about lovemaking. After a while, that becomes normal. The sex life disintegrates, taking with it the good part of life that we are working so hard to achieve.

That is a much bigger problem than the medical community or the media will acknowledge. Research from universities in Great Britain and the United States[5] reveals that reports of activities indicating sexual satisfaction—frequent kissing, cuddling, caressing, and concern for your own and your partner's orgasm—signaled greater relationship happiness and better health. In other words, good sex is good for us. By that logic, bad sex (or no sex) is bad for us.

I believe another reason sex has become less frequent and less satisfying is the poor sex education in this country. For years, many schools, communities, and parents have chosen to give their children minimal information about sexuality and no information at all about subjects including erectile dysfunction, the orgasm, or the differences between how men and women desire and experience sex.

When that happens, young people get most of their sexual education from peers, some magazines, and pornography but not from authorities. Yet somehow, with this fragmented and inaccurate information, they are expected to know and understand their own sexuality, not to mention the sexuality of their partners. Such understanding is unlikely to be achieved under these circumstances. Therefore, as a result of our broken sex-education system, we have produced a generation of men and women who are sexually deficient and sexually ignorant. Myths are filling the gaps. Many parts of the sexual experience that couples encounter when they spend years together—ED in the man, low libido in the woman, for instance—are very common and treatable but are regarded as surprises and catastrophes. Ignorance is *not* sexual bliss.

Here is one example. Among my patients were a forty-eight-year-old man and his wife, who was forty-three. They had been married for eighteen years. I treated them for medical issues including high blood pressure and acid reflux. She had a hysterectomy at a younger age for a fibroid tumor, and therefore they have no children. They both work and seem happy and attached to each other. But they don't exercise and are overweight. They both drink two to three glasses of wine during dinner, and I was surprised when they told me that they could only remember having sex two or three times during the last year. I asked about performance problems, and they could not think of any. So why did this young couple not have sex? They said, "We just don't think about it. We come home from work, eat dinner, read the paper, watch TV, and go to bed."

I have encountered many couples like this husband and wife—in particular after the kids have left the house. I think what is happening to these couples is a symbol of the boring lifestyle many people choose to live. Because they were never educated about sex, they never experimented and found out how enjoyable it is. It's like never seeing a rainbow or trying honey; you don't know what you're missing. I encouraged the couple to return to an active sex life as a reward for exercise. I also asked them to cut back on the alcohol.

Six months later, they reported that they had changed their lifestyle. They were walking together three to four miles daily, drinking alcohol only socially with friends, and had each lost more than ten pounds. As for sexual activity, they said, "Yes, we really enjoy sex now."

It didn't take me much time to help change this couple's life, but why didn't they think about that themselves? We have made sex an optional part of a healthy life, and it is not. It is essential.

MEDICINE DOESN'T RESPECT SEX

THE MEMBERS OF MY PROFESSION certainly bear some of the blame for these problems. By and large, the medical profession looks at sex only as it relates to things like sexually transmitted diseases, prostate disorders, birth control, menstrual disorders, and menopause. Few doctors think about healthy sexual function and a fulfilling sex life as being part of their patients' overall wellness picture. Is it any wonder that only about 4 percent of patients bring up sexual problems with their primary care physicians?[6] And more troubling, even this low percentage will never get sympathy or any practical help from the physician. In my career, I have seldom had a patient bring up sexuality as a topic for discussion; patients only responded to my initiating questions.

Modern medicine has extended life expectancy, cured disease, and turned death sentences like AIDS into chronic but manageable conditions, but the profession hasn't evolved with the times to address the importance of sexuality as part of overall wellness. It turns out that intimacy and happiness are just as important to well-being and longevity as a healthy heart and well-managed blood sugar. For example, research shows that there is a strong association between sexual dysfunction and depression in both men and women.[7] On the other side, good sex appears to boost the immune system, lower blood pressure, reduce pain, reduce the risk of cardiovascular disease, and improve sleep, and it may help men avoid prostate cancer.[8]

As many diseases that were common until the late twentieth century have retreated in the face of vaccines and better public sanitation, medicine has failed to adapt to today's society. Patients tend to be more sedentary now, and because they have access to limitless medical information that is not always correct, they are more anxious, and they want communication and connection with their healthcare providers. However, physicians are not providing that intimacy.

The profession has become less about healing and more about record keeping, using blood tests, MRIs, and CT scans, or prescribing medications and avoiding legal liability.

People go online to find medical information and often come to their appointments armed with facts and ideas about their health, many of which are wrong. Still, physicians feel pressured to have all the answers instead of admitting they don't know the answer and being willing to learn from their interaction with the patient. The entire system encourages medicine to be mechanical, faceless, cold, and dissatisfying, once again ignoring the emotional side of wellness.

There is also a medicolegal system that holds the threat of litigation and financial ruin over physicians' heads, forcing them to avoid deviating from the standard protocol, to order unnecessary tests, and to emphasize lengthy documentation for fear of being sued. The legal system has made some physicians paranoid about their own patients suing them, making them practice based only on the standards and written protocols that will help them avoid legal action. That removes the talent, skill, and intuition from medicine. It is an art, and too many physicians practice it today as a science.

Unfortunately, medicine knows only a small piece of how the miraculous human body works and reacts, so it is essential that the doctor use common sense, judgment, experience, and gut instinct in treating patients. When the physician is forced to act like a machine or computer program, that's gone. He or she ends up practicing only defensive medicine, which hurts the patient and often leads to mistakes that end up resulting in lawsuits anyway. That is one of the reasons the United States spends more per capita on health care than any other developed country[9] and yet has millions of people not covered by health insurance.

PHYSICIANS ARE NOT BEING ALLOWED TO PRACTICE MEDICINE

MORE PHYSICIANS AND PATIENTS MUST learn and accept the fact that physicians are not being allowed to practice medicine. Right now, we have a "disease care" system, not a health-care system. Physicians and laypeople have become convinced that medicine should be about preventing disease, when in reality it should be about feeling vibrant, healthy, and happy. By that definition, wellness includes the satisfaction and enjoyment of a great sex life and a strong relationship!

However, our system currently rewards doctors who treat their practices like conveyor belts: patients sign in and enter through one door, then exit through another door an hour later, perhaps with a prescription in hand, having spent maybe fifteen minutes with the doctor. It's just as likely they will have seen a physician assistant or nurse practitioner. There is nothing wrong with those professions, but the simple fact that so many doctors rely on them sends a terrible message: *It doesn't matter who you see because you're not getting individualized care anyway.*

The other problem is the poor communication with the clinic or the doctor's office. Most of the time when you call the doctor's office, there will not be a person to answer you. Instead, you will get a telephone system telling you which numbers to push and to "leave a massage, and we will call you back." If you are lucky, you will get a call back the next day. If your problem cannot wait, you are forced to go to the emergency room and spend hours waiting, ending up with a fat bill that may not be covered by your insurance. When you add in the cost of medical insurance and bureaucracy designed to hinder care for the sake of saving money, what you have is a broken system.

To me, as much as I love what I do, that is the wrong message to send. No wonder patients feel like they're being given a pill and sent on their way—that's what is happening! This approach reflects the fundamental flaw at the heart of the way we practice medicine today, which is that physicians are expected to *treat disease but not necessarily prevent it and definitely not promote health.* If your physician were really intent on helping you stay healthy, he would be talking to you not only about your sex life and your stress levels, but also about nutrition, exercise, sleep, and more. Instead, in a typical physical, the PCP (or usually his assistant) takes a medical history, checks your blood pressure, listens to your heart, looks at your skin to check for anything that could be precancerous, palpates your abdomen looking for anything unusual, and looks in your eyes, ears, and throat. And that's about it. You give blood at a lab and get a few numbers back that show your cholesterol level, blood sugar, and so on.

If your cholesterol is high, the doctor might prescribe a statin; if your blood pressure is elevated, he might put you on an ACE inhibitor. That's it. No attention is paid to the person, just the symptoms. Even depression or anxiety are treated as conditions that will be addressed with medication.

Most doctors don't practice medicine this way because they like it. They do it because they have no other choice. If they want to get reimbursed by the insurance companies, they have to play by their rules. Not only are the typical PCPs incentivized to keep costs down for insurers, they are also forced to prescribe meds that are least expensive but not necessarily the best for the patient. Forget about counseling a patient who's prediabetic to exercise and lose forty pounds; just give the patient metformin and move on.

Insurance companies are aware that the average person stays with a given employer for about two years. Since most people get their health insurance through their employers, the insurance companies have no incentive to spend money on preventive medicine, early disease detection, or wellness because they know that within a year or two, that patient will be a client of another insurer. Their interest is in treating current symptoms and keeping costs down. That will be conveyed to the physician who works for them. Obviously, there will be a conflict of interest between the patient's needs and the needs of insurance company's stockholders, and the physician is caught between them.

Here is an example of how it works. My patient, a fifty-eight-year-old man in good health, had gallstones. I sent him to a surgeon to have his gallbladder removed in order to prevent infection and rupture. The insurance company declined to approve the surgery.

Two years later while he was on a cruise with his wife in South America, his gallbladder became infected, the ship's doctor didn't handle the problem immediately, and the organ ruptured. It took another two days to get him to a hospital where he survived but wound up hospitalized for four months. The insurance company that paid those treatment bills was different from the one that declined his preventive surgery, so I guess the first insurer made the correct decision, right?

There are four other main reasons that the majority of PCPs don't bring up the subject of sexuality with their patients as part of routine physicals:

1. They are not trained to believe that there's any connection between sexual performance and sexuality and physical and mental health. In medical school they focus exclusively on STDs and sexual dysfunction as symptoms of underlying illness such as cardiovascular disease. Sexuality as an entity is completely ignored, as is the role of happiness and contentment in wellness. But who could deny that being happy and feeling content are parts of leading a full, healthy life?

2. Physicians are not trained to handle sexual dysfunction in the context of a relationship and will usually refer such matters to someone like a sex therapist, urologist, or gynecologist, just to avoid handling this topic. They may not want to discuss or talk with the patient about sex as they feel embarrassed, which is a human response but has no place in the work of medical professionals. Imagine a urologist telling a male patient that he doesn't want to check him for prostate cancer because sticking his finger in

the patient's behind embarrasses him! The patient would rightly be outraged.

Any patient has the right to expect the physician to be, if not comfortable, at least professional in discussing matters related to sexual activity. For one thing, sexual dysfunction can be the result of treatable medical conditions and can also impact mental health, which is in the physician's purview. "It makes the doctor squeamish" is no excuse for not talking about sex and not training physicians to discuss it intelligently.

3. The medical world has created an impersonal environment where there is little trust. Sexuality is already a topic with a social stigma attached to it, and when we herd people into an office like cattle, we make them even less likely to open up to us about such intimate topics. That is why we will talk about our acid reflux disease, hemorrhoids, bowel and bladder function, vaginal bleeding, and on and on, but when it comes to sexual function, that's personal and off limits. Physicians are not creating a "safe space" for sexuality in their offices.

4. Recently, fears of sexual harassment have complicated things, mostly for male doctors and female patients. Now liability insurance companies instruct male physicians to have a nurse present with them at all times when they are with female patients. What if the patient wants to discuss intimate or personal issues without the presence of a third person in the room?

WHY I DON'T HAVE ANYONE ELSE IN THE ROOM

THESE ARE SOME OF THE MANY REASONS that in my medical practice, I defy conventional wisdom by allowing no one but myself and the patient in the room during my examination and conversation, except during a procedure when I need help or when I am doing a pelvic examination.

I want my office and exam room to be a place where my patients can share the most intimate parts of their lives, including their fears and anxieties, without fear of being judged. I need them to trust me and open up about the most intimate parts of their lives because only when I know everything that is happening can I identify possible causes for their distress and recommend solutions. Having someone else in the room destroys that sense of intimacy and trust and discourages patients from opening their hearts and talking about what really bothers them, including sex and sexual relations.

Look at it this way: If I have someone else in the room to make sure I am not doing something inappropriate to my patients, what message does that send? First, it is a clear demonstration to the patient that I am not trustworthy. It also says that my utmost concern is to protect myself, and that is not why people go to their physician. They come to me because they know that in that moment my only concern is them and their well-being.

This is vitally important because between 75 and 90 percent of the reasons that people see their PCP are related to the effects of chronic stress, from high blood pressure and skin conditions to depression and anxiety.[11] I know that seems very high, but it's true. Many Americans are unhealthy—overweight, consuming bad food, not exercising, and neglecting their health by smoking and drinking. Frequently, their medical conditions are associated with anxiety and depression, but the patient will not know the association, so they may see the doctor for one symptom and discover another problem they knew nothing about.

The same is true when a sexual problem is the culprit of his symptoms. Someone suffering from headaches, depression, and heart palpitations caused by the stress of a troubled marriage and frustrating sex life won't be helped by a fifteen-minute exam and a pill. That person will be helped by a caring physician who listens, earns trust, and respects the person, not just the symptoms. This actually would lower the cost of medical care, as treatment can be straightforward without the cost of unnecessary specialists and tests.

One of the reasons my patients keep coming to me—and recommending new patients who keep me busy and happily working—is that they love the private, intimate, trusting nature of that unhurried time together. During my forty-five years, I have never heard complaints from any patient about not having someone else in the room or experienced any unwillingness expressed by patients to partner with my approach.

BEING OPEN WITH YOUR PHYSICIAN ABOUT YOUR FEARS

My patient, a thirty-two-year-old woman, made an appointment to see me, telling my nurse that she was suffering from back pain. When I saw her, I asked her how long she'd had this back pain, and she responded that the back pain was not bothering her anymore. I was puzzled, and then she said that her main concern was a recurrence of her genital herpes. She had never told her husband about it because she was afraid that he would reject her. That was also why she was so secretive with my nurse.

Examining a lesion on her thigh, I confirmed that it was genital herpes and treated it accordingly. However, knowing that she was concerned for her marriage, I discussed this with her. I suggested that she and her husband come and see me together, and when they did, I explained this common infection and told them that many couples manage to live normal and happy lives—including sex lives—along with healthy children. Her husband's main concern was her safety and her health, and he was eager to help. I believe the conversation helped this couple keep their marriage and happiness intact.

FOUR LAYPERSON
MISUNDERSTANDINGS ABOUT SEX

IT IS UNFAIR TO LAY the American attitudes about sexuality solely at the feet of physicians and the medical community. Men and women laypeople are just as responsible for the suppression of this important conversation and for making sex a topic more likely to lead to shame, discomfort, or laughter than compassion and understanding.

If we dig into the data about American attitudes toward sexuality, we find some disturbing trends that contribute to the problems I'm talking about. In 2014, the American Sexual Health Association conducted a survey of more than three thousand American adults who were in a committed relationship and dealing with at least one sexual-health-related issue.[12] They found that while 64 percent believed that their sex life influenced their overall satisfaction with their lives, only 38 percent were actually satisfied with their sex lives.

Only one out of four respondents felt they could be honest with their partners regarding sexual problems. Women's and men's priorities were completely different, too: men's main focus was on the physical ability to perform and on experimentation in the bedroom, while women were more interested in achieving orgasm, bonding emotionally, and enjoying sex. Finally, a third of the people surveyed were resigned to having a worse sex life in twenty years, despite knowing that sex was important to their health and happiness.

That is a tragedy. How does such a deep disconnect happen? The answer is misinformation and fear. Because Americans do not have a longstanding tradition of talking openly about sex in raising their children, men and women reach adulthood thinking that they can't talk about sex even with their partners. They talk past the subject, and as a result, stay undercover and live with falsehoods and anxiety about the subject when they could simply get it out in the open and resolve so much by better communication. People hide from their partners and never discuss sexuality with them, even though they may be with them for many years. Parents will not show sexual affection to each other in the presence of their children, and they often avoid conversations with their kids about sex. Children see this behavior and model it. The entire subject becomes taboo.

Let me tell you about the dynamic that I have seen over and over again in my office. A man or woman will come to see me about some health question that, on the surface, is unrelated to sexuality, such as high blood pressure or cholesterol. During the course of our private conversation, I will ask about his or her sexual relations. If there is a problem in that area, the patient will often show great distress. When I ask more questions, I often hear a variation of "I haven't ever spoken to my husband/wife about this." I cannot count how many times patients have confessed to me their fear, embarrassment, sadness, resentment, or anger about a poor sex life while telling me that they have never shared a word with their partners.

That is the biggest problem we face in solving the issue of unsatisfying sex and broken relationships. Without communication, there is no real intimacy. There always will be an unknown secret between them, even if they lived together for many years. Without intimacy, there can be no sexual satisfaction in the long term. How can we know what our partners need and how to please them if we are not talking with them about what they like and dislike and the challenges they may be experiencing sexually?

How can we let our partners know about our own sexual issues and expect them to help us address them without communication? We need to teach people to talk to their partners and learn more about the physiology and psychology of sex—and particularly how sexuality differs strongly in men and women.

Americans suffer from four important misconceptions about sex that create this crisis:

1. **We treat sex as a luxury.** In *The Atlantic*, journalist Kate Julian wrote, "Most people need jobs; that's not the case with relationships and sex."[13] That is simply wrong. Sex is not a luxury; it is a necessity of a whole and healthy life. We are far too cavalier about the importance of sexual satisfaction and its benefits:

    » stronger intimacy and bonding in a relationship
    » greater feelings of well-being. In 2017, psychologist Anik Debrot and her colleagues found that sexual activity promotes affection, which, in turn, promotes well-being[14]
    » relief from stress, anxiety, and insomnia
    » a more positive body image and healthy habits

    In addition, a 2014 study found a strong correlation between a couple's sexual activity, marital happiness, and good health.[15] Sexuality also creates ambition and self-confidence. And sexuality motivates a person to push hard to achieve goals.

    There are many more examples from research showing the clear link between a satisfying sex life, strong relationships, and positive physical and mental health. Sex is not something we can take or leave; it is an integral part of our lives and important for a positive outcome.

2. **We assume that everyone should be naturally good at sex.** There is a belief that people are either good at sex or not good at it. Also, we tend to believe that there is only one kind of being "good" at sex—which, for men, usually involves being able to have intercourse and maintain an erection for a long time before climax. These are ideas that have nothing to do with reality.

The truth is that no one is naturally perfect at sex, and there are many ways to be good at it. Each of us has to learn how to do the things that bring satisfaction to our partners and to teach our partners what brings us satisfaction. But doing that means communicating about sex and talking honestly about what we like and do not like. Over time, and with practice, we can and do become "better" at sex when emotionally inhibiting factors like fear, guilt, and embarrassment are removed. Also, there are many ways to be "good" at sexual performance. What matters most is what you and your partner like and want, and that can change and be better achieved over time. Each couple is different and gets satisfaction differently.

The important thing to remember is that not feeling like you are adept at sex probably has less to do with your physical prowess and more to do with fear, lack of information, and factors like hormone levels and emotions. You can always learn and improve your sexual function and ability, but only if you talk about it and share with your partner.

3. **We assume our sexuality will not change over time.** Couples know that their bodies will age and they will likely gain weight, develop wrinkles, and experience other normal changes over time. That is all part of the normal process of living. But couples seem to have a blind spot regarding changes in libido, arousal, performance, and orgasm. So many of us assume that sex will be the same when we are seventy years old as it was when we were thirty years old. This creates another taboo within the bounds of the relationship and also creates false and damaging expectations. Just as the weather changes, you can expect changes in your partner, so you will need to talk to him or her and adapt to those changes.

Sex will not remain the same as we age because we don't remain the same. That doesn't mean that sex cannot continue and cannot be good; research shows that as we age, many of us continue to enjoy great, satisfying sex. One poll found that among men and women between sixty-five and eighty years old, 40 percent were still having sex—54 percent if they were in steady relationships.[16] So the idea that people past retirement age are asexual is false.

However, there are changes. Everything, from vaginal dryness and uterine prolapse in women to ED and enlarged prostate in men can make sex more challenging, but if both partners want to continue having good sex into their sixties, seventies, and beyond, there is a way to get around every challenge. I personally believe that sexuality in humans never dies; it can only be extinguished by ignorance.

4. **We assume that men's and women's sexuality—and the roles of men and women in sexual satisfaction—are identical.** Understanding that men and women do not experience sexuality in the same way or derive pleasure from sex in all the same ways is the key insight here. Men's pleasure in sex, as we will discuss later, always revolves around the orgasm. If the man does not climax, he considers the sexual encounter to have been a waste and is unsatisfied. On the other hand, research shows that women do not always climax during any kind of sex, even during masturbation, but that the woman's pleasure from the sexual act also comes from intimacy and satisfying her partner. The needs of the two genders are very different, making it dangerous to impose one's needs on the other.

Men's and women's roles in sex are also very different. Men are usually the pursuers, while women are more often in the position to acquiesce to men's advances for sex. We attach shame to these realities instead of accepting that they are BOTH right; they are simply the ways genders work together. If we fail to acknowledge these differences, we might shame the man for needing sex when it's simply his biology talking. If we go too far to the other extreme, we can accept the man's natural desire to have multiple women at his call to be used for sex without intimacy, which is exploitation.

On the other side, without clear communication and understanding, it is easy for a woman to feel that by giving into the man's need for sex when she doesn't desire sex herself, she is being used, when in reality, sex is just as beneficial for her as for him.

Let me be clear. Across the board, men and women in this culture make groundless assumptions about sexuality that have no basis in fact. These can easily be countered by communication and education, and should be. Doing so would prevent damaging misunderstandings that hurt feelings, harm relationships, and leave people believing that they have no alternative but to endure a lifetime of poor sex.

> I've noticed through my observations that while adult men know very little about the sexual physiology and emotions of women, women are even worse. Two ladies are talking about male sexuality, passions, and performance, and one asks the other, "I wonder what men say about women and sex when we're not around?"
>
> The second woman says, "I can tell you what they talk about with each other—the same things we women talk about."
>
> The first lady gasps and says, "Oh my God, I never knew they were that dirty!"

THE DAMAGE DONE BY SEXUAL IGNORANCE

TELEVISION, MOVIES, NEWSPAPERS, magazines, the Internet—the media do not use sex as a tool for education and good health but instead for sensational news and as a way to smear people for bad behavior and discrimination. This creates a negative stigma around sex, contributing to the shame. The negative impact of media contributes to our inability to talk about and candidly deal with sexual dissatisfaction and ignorance, which powerfully affects three major areas of life: marriage, physical well-being, and mental health.

Marriage. There are many reasons why couples break up, but one of the leading reasons is always a change in the pattern of sexual activity. Sometimes, one person wants more sex than the other partner is willing to provide, while other times, one partner has neglected to take care of himself or herself, leading to diminished physical attraction and depression. I have seen this so many times with the patients who come into my office. They are desperate, frustrated, angry, and resigned, convinced that they need to leave the marriage to find the sex lives they feel they deserve. Of course, before it gets to this point, it will take a long and agonizing course of bad feeling, loss of sleep, and waste of energy. The culprit of the conflict may be sex, but it can snowball into something worse, like verbal abuse, alcohol use, or violence.

That word *deserve* may be the key here. It is not only the absence of sex that kills marriages but the feeling that your partner has given up on the marriage and on you. That can ruin relationships. Remember, sexual activity correlates strongly with intimacy and communication, so a sexless marriage (which psychologists define as the couple having sex ten or fewer times in a year) can send the message that one partner doesn't care about intimacy or communication—or doesn't care about you.

Infidelity is another common result of sexual dissatisfaction with a partner. Most infidelity comes from men, and it's a major cause of divorce. But we can see why in the difference in sexuality between men and women. While the woman by nature seeks intimacy, deep feeling, and closeness from sex, the man's sexual desire is driven by a powerful urge and the desire for orgasm. This makes him less emotional and more impulsive, more likely to pursue sex outside his marriage. I have seen many men engaging in infidelity in a moment of sexual excitement and soon after regretting it. For the woman, this is an emotional trauma and insult that often cannot be repaired.

Despite all this, people may be reluctant to admit that a lack of sex has contributed to the damage to their marriage, but it's still likely to be partially responsible. A 2015 study from *Social Psychological and Personality Science*, in which more than thirty thousand Americans were interviewed over four decades, found that married couples who had sex at least once a week were happier than those who didn't.[17] A study by a British law firm also found that sexual problems were the most common factor in divorce cases, being involved in 43 percent.[18] Sex matters, even if we don't like to talk about it.

Physical well-being. Let's look at one very important area of health that can be improved by sex: cardiovascular health. Sexual activity improves circulation and motivates us to exercise, eat a healthy diet, and pay better attention to our appearance and lifestyle.

Sex is exercise, and exercise is good for the heart, for both women and men. One study[19] found that men in their fifties who have sex at least twice a week find their risk of heart disease reduced by 45 percent, compared with men who have sex less often. Also, since stress is a major contributor to heart disease and sex is a wonderful stress reducer, regular sex can help prevent heart disease by reducing the impact of chronic stress.

Lack of good sex, on the other hand, can both contribute to heart disease by allowing stress to rage unchecked and indicate potential heart disease, as damaged arteries can lead to issues like ED or poor vaginal lubrication.

Mental health. One Chinese study[20] found that more frequent sex led to greater overall happiness, which is not surprising when you consider that frequent sex is usually a sign of a strong relationship. Counselors also say that sexual frustration can be a harbinger of other deeper emotions like fear or pain and, if left unchecked, could lead to clinical depression and other problems.[21] So while the lack of sex or bad sex on its own might not *cause* mental illness, it can be a sign of deeper issues that should be addressed.

WHAT CAN WE DO?

IN THE END, FREQUENT and mutually-satisfying sex is good for individuals, marriages, and society. So how do we remedy the fear, shame, taboo, and lack of communication that presents itself in my office on a daily basis when I see a husband or wife near tears with anger and frustration? We begin, I believe, by bringing the physician into the equation as an objective third party.

I understand that many doctors will not be pleased at the idea of becoming "sex therapists" for their patients, but this is part of their responsibility and something they need to become comfortable with, just like checking a patient's blood pressure or pulse. Patients who struggle with the emotional baggage of sexual problems often need a third party to step in when emotions are running high and objectivity is needed. They are at a loss, as they don't realize how often their medical disorders are connected to their sexual problems and the underlying stress, and they don't know how to address those problems.

I want to see PCPs talking about sexuality as part of routine annual checkups—bringing up sexual satisfaction and performance not as aspects of possible disease, but as parts of their patients' overall happiness. As I mentioned before, our medical and social systems cannot continue to ignore this basic human biological need without serious consequences. Medical technology will never substitute for a caring physician who asks good questions, listens, builds trust, and offers sound, objective advice.

Here's an example of the kind of negative social impact I'm talking about. In modern cities, city planners and engineers have given us public transit systems, parks, hospitals, fire stations, electrical grids, clean water, wireless Internet—a host of wonderful essentials. However, most cities overlook a basic but critical human need: public toilets. This causes tremendous harm and suffering to the entire population. When I discussed this issue with people, they told me that when no toilets are available, they avoid drinking water in order to avoid the need to go to bathroom!

This will have negative ramifications for their health: dehydration, fatigue, muscle cramps, headaches, and even kidney stones and infection. Women endure serious discomfort during their monthly cycles to the point that they avoid going into the city for work or pleasure. Older people with enlarged prostate and bladder problems also suffer from the lack of facilities. And in cities like San Francisco and Los Angeles, the streets are contaminated with human feces and urine from the many homeless, creating an enormous heath risk.

My point is that in overlooking something that seems humble and ordinary, in not giving it the respect it is due, society has created a huge problem. It is the same with sexuality. And I believe the solution starts with physicians. Physicians who ask good questions and listen with respect will find their patients opening up to them in unprecedented ways. After I spoke to my patients about sex, many told me that it was the first time they had ever been asked such questions by any physician. It broke the taboo for them and encouraged them to talk to me, to see me as their partner. No one ever complained that my questions were too intrusive, inappropriate, or irrelevant. No one ever declined to discuss the topic.

Couples must also get in the habit of talking openly to each other, lovingly and without judgment, about their sexuality—likes, dislikes, fantasies, fetishes, fears, physical issues, everything. Nothing should be off limits. These conversations can be done gradually, working up to more intimate matters. But I know from experience with my patients that the more couples communicate openly and compassionately, the stronger their bond—and usually, the better their sexual experience.

OPEN DISCUSSIONS ABOUT
SEX CAN RESTORE HAPPINESS
AND REUNITE COUPLES

Another couple I had treated for several years were in their mid-sixties and had been married for thirty-five years. But now they both seemed unhappy and were struggling with various symptoms. They were living separate lives and sleeping in separate rooms. I saw them in separate appointments and was astonished to hear different stories from them in response to the same questions.

The man said that they slept in different rooms because the woman did not respond to his sexual advances, and that upset him. The woman said that they slept in separate rooms because he snored at night and moved a lot. He told me that the last time they had sex was two years earlier; she said that they had sex two or three times a month and she was fine with that, but she was upset that her husband didn't make advances and showed no interest in her. That made her feel like he didn't care.

Much of the time, lying and miscommunication are the problem when it comes to sex. The different stories made me ask more questions, and after more exploration, the wife admitted to me that she sometimes had low libido and was not always ready to have sex but felt uncomfortable admitting that. She also told me that her husband frequently had problems with sexual performance but would not talk about it.

I have found this in many, many couples. Men and women pass guilt onto their partner, report inaccurate information, and refuse to openly discuss problems with each other, all because of embarrassment. They don't intend to lie, and I am not a judge in sex court! But they do lie, and that only makes it harder to find solutions.

Finally, I managed to talk with both of them together and gently discussed what they did not know about low libido and ED. It made sense to them, and it did not take much effort on my part to get them talking to each other about sex and helping one another. When I saw them in following visits, they had already changed their lifestyle. They had gone back to having sexual relations twice a week and were enjoying it. They were not using two bedrooms anymore and joked about being able to have guests over because they had a guest room again.

Chapter Two

FORTY-FIVE YEARS OF TREATING A SILENT EPIDEMIC

You might think I am exaggerating the impact of sexual dysfunction and lack of communication about sex on health and happiness, but I am not. Nearly every day, I encounter patients who are suffering because of the stress, shame, and secrecy that surround their sex lives, which results in marital troubles, family strife, and health disorders. These are just a few examples that show the human tragedy of our poor education, cultural taboos, and lack of information.

A nice couple, the kind of people others in our society envy, came to my office. The man was fifty-two years old, educated, professional, healthy, and good-looking and apparently devoted to his family. His wife was fifty-one, charming, and educated, with a good career. They had married twenty-six years earlier and raised three beautiful kids who graduated college.

I had known these people for many years, and as their last child left to go to college, I expected to see a happy couple looking forward to years of good times and freedom together. Instead, I saw pain. While the husband was active and exercised, his wife kept complaining of multiple somatic symptoms, which necessitated numerous medical tests and visits to specialists with no relief. The man was very supportive and accompanied her throughout the stressful process.

Recently, the husband had approached his wife to tell her that he wanted to dissolve their marriage. When she asked why now, he told her that he had been thinking about it for some time but was waiting for their last child to leave the house. She admitted that she didn't understand the reason for his decision, and she was in a great deal of distress and emotional pain. But because they had both been my patients, I knew what she did not know. Her husband had told me what the problem was: a sexless marriage.

Over the years, when I saw the husband for regular physicals, he told me about the problems at home and eventually about his plan. He explained very clearly that he had put up with this situation during those long years because he loved his kids. Yes, he loved his wife, too, but he could never talk to her about sex. He would not have sex with other women because it would be against his conscience but instead relieved his urges, reluctantly, through masturbation. Now he had given up. He had no reason to continue with the marriage.

I asked the wife about their intimate relations, and her response was that for the past fifteen years they didn't have any sexual relations at all. She explained that she was too occupied by her medical issues and raising children and felt no sexual desire. For a time, her husband tried to coax her into sexual activity, but soon after, he withdrew and never approached her sexually again, although he continued his devotion to his family.

At this point, she told me that she had begun to lose her identity as a feminine wife and attractive woman. She sank into anxiety, depression, and fear, which resulted in more symptoms and multiple visits to doctors to "fix" symptoms that were clearly caused by emotional and mental stress. It surprised me that this woman, as intelligent and professional as she was, could not figure out what was happening. Perhaps it is human nature that when we are preoccupied, we become blind to what is right in front of us.

I asked her about what happened between her and her husband, and her story matched his in many ways. I explained the importance of sex for both men and women in a strong, healthy relationship. After my explanation, I asked her whether she thought the fifteen years of sexual drought could have caused the breakup of her marriage. She expressed astonishment and then said, "Why didn't he tell me? Nobody told me!" and burst into tears. It was a heartbreaking scene, made worse by the fact that things had gone too far. The marriage was over, and there was no going back.

Ironically, her husband and I had both tried to discuss sex with her over the years, but every time she would brush the question aside and insist that everything was fine. She had adopted denial as a way of escaping her reality. By the way, all her medical symptoms were also related to that loss of identity as a loving, sexual woman.

In the end, she spent many thousands of dollars on unnecessary doctor visits and lost her marriage.

The question is, did it have to end that way? And the answer is absolutely NOT. The distorted sexual system many people are locked into and the secrecy, denial, and lack of knowledge and communication that system fosters are to blame.

———

I SAW A WOMAN IN MY OFFICE, fifty-six years old, intelligent, and professional. Her husband, fifty-eight, was also a successful professional. They had been married for twenty-eight years and raised two children, now grown. But for the previous two years, the woman had struggled with a facial rash and acne. She had seen more than ten specialists and received many different medical treatments. The problem was that after the lesions healed partially, they would return and become active again. Consequently, the woman's life changed. She would not go out in public because she was embarrassed. She became devastated and depressed because of her facial acne and some scar tissue.

Her husband was devoted to her, but for the previous two years, he had not approached her sexually. She said that he had stopped looking at her completely, even when she walked in the room naked just to attract his attention. After having great sex an average of three times a week in the past, they'd had two years without any sex at all. She came to feel that her husband was not coming to her because of her face, saying, "With a face like mine, who wants to look at me?" It was terrible and sad.

Her sex drive remained strong, but she felt abandoned and

unwanted. Her recurrent acne suggested to me that her sex drive would be strong because acne is usually the result of a hormonal surge that stimulates the oily glands in the skin to produce excess oil and become inflamed. And when the sex drive is not satisfied, as we see with teenagers, those hormone levels remain high and the acne continues unabated.

Still, I was perplexed about her self-image and her depression over her life, which seemed strange for a woman who was truly very charming and attractive. I took the conversation back to both hers and her husband's sex life and asked whether she recalled how her husband's sexual performance had been and whether he had started to experience difficulties when her acne problems started two years ago. She recalled a few incidents of him having difficulty performing back then, but he never discussed it and seemed to brush it off as unimportant, and she never connected it with his sexual withdrawal from her.

I explained to her the impact that ED can have on a man. Men, feeling emasculated, can become anxious, nervous, filled with shame, and helpless, not knowing how to respond or handle the problem. Many men hide from their partners in order to conceal what they see as weakness and failure. I suggested to the woman that her husband had experienced, two years previously, one incident of ED and ever since had felt terrible shame. I said, "Your husband started to hide what he saw as his failure from you and from himself by avoiding sex. The more you tried to bring him to the arena, the more he has kept his distance."

Her face lit up. She understood and agreed that this was the obscured issue. I had seen her husband a few times before, but each time he brushed aside the issue of any problem with his performance and didn't acknowledge his sexual difficulties. He was ashamed to talk about it, yet he asked me for a prescription for Viagra. You can see how horrendous the effect of ED was on the man, his wife, and their life together. I have no doubt that her unsatisfied sex drive was contributing to her acne, which fueled the cycle. She left the office begging me to help her husband, but something more important took place in our conversation: she got correct information about what was happening in her personal life. That single conversation changed her entire perception of herself, her marriage, her husband, and her future.

In my following meeting with her husband, we had an open conversation, during which time he finally opened his heart and expressed his shame. Now he was ready to listen, and with his wife's cooperation and my encouragement, he overcome the fear and was able to function as normally as before. Their sexual activities, intimacy, and love returned.

It is hard to believe how often sexual problems can be resolved and life can be improved by direct and open conversation.

———

A FORTY-NINE-YEAR-OLD MAN CAME TO me to check the health of his heart. He had three children and had been married to what he described as a "hot-blooded" Spanish woman for twenty-five years. He hadn't seen any doctor in the past ten years, which is more common for men than for women. When he last saw a physician, he was told that he had an enlarged heart, and he also experienced some degree of ED for the first time. This is not unusual; some people with heart problems become fearful of having sex because they are afraid they will have a heart attack, which is extremely rare.

The diagnosis of an enlarged heart was traumatic for this young man, and it scared him out of seeing any doctor for either his ED or his heart condition. Afraid of what he might learn about his heart, and embarrassed by his ED, he neglected both issues and entered into denial. During the next ten years, he suffered immensely and tried to avoid sexual contact, and yet he tried diligently to satisfy his wife sexually, either by manual stimulation or by attempting intercourse with her using Viagra, despite his fear.

Finally, he came to see me. I heard his story during our long conversation, and during my examination, I found nothing medically wrong with him . . . including his heart! The doctor he had seen ten years before had been wrong. He had suffered needlessly. I told him that in my opinion, all his sexual problems were related to the poor communication with his previous physician and his fear of a condition that he did not have. He was very happy and felt reinvigorated. His fear gradually dissipated, and his vigorous drive and ambitions came back. He carried Cialis with him to help with sex with his wife, but rarely used it.

Fear can cause people to hide from a devil that doesn't even exist. It's incredible how a simple open conversation between patient and physician can dispel those fears and set the patient free.

———

ANOTHER CASE INVOLVES AN EIGHTY-YEAR-OLD MAN and his sixty-five-year-old wife, who were both my patients. Until twelve years ago, they had a good sex life. Then she went into menopause, and her sexual behavior changed. She lost all interest in sex, declined any sex with her husband, and would not even talk with him about this topic.

They became estranged over this. He acted impatiently and abrasively out of sexual frustration and the sense that she no longer cared about him or their relationship. His wife grew angry at his behavior, thinking that he was being unreasonable to desire sex when she didn't want to have it, and believing that her decisions about sex were her prerogative and affected her alone. Their relationship became superficial—they would show up for activities with friends, but there was no intimacy or emotional affection between them. The husband was candid with me about all this, including the fact that he had started having extramarital relations. In his seventies, he remained sexually active with the help of Viagra.

During those same years, his wife struggled, experiencing poor sleep, low energy and motivation, and depression, which led to many doctor visits. They were basically living two separate lives and did not have a marriage at all. During my individual encounter with her during her physical examination to evaluate her somatic symptoms, we started to discuss her attitude and approach toward her intimate life with her husband. She expressed to me that since her libido was low and she lost her sexual desire, she elected to have no sexual contact with her husband. She allowed her actions to be driven by her libido, without consideration for the potential ramifications to herself or her marriage. I brought to her attention that sexual activity is a positive physiological function and was good for her own health and well-being. It would revitalize her sense of femininity, desirability, and attractiveness and buoy her self-esteem and feelings of self-worth, thereby leading to an abatement of many of her somatic symptoms. Additionally, it would definitely bring her husband closer to her and make him a happier and more pleasant partner, which would lead to a harmonious marriage and happier family life. She said that nobody ever brought this to her attention, and she appreciated this new perspective and was very open to making the appropriate changes for her well-being and seemingly important marriage.

When he came to see me in my office for his yearly physical four months later, I noticed that at eighty years old he was happy, invigorated, motivated, and healthy. At the conclusion of the exam and meeting, I offered him his usual prescription for Viagra, but this time he surprised me by declining it. I thought first that he had stopped sexual activity altogether, but I was astonished to hear that his wife had made a complete turnaround after my conversation with her. They were back to having sex once a week.

Now they love each other more than ever before, spend more time together, exercise together, and are very happy. I asked him if he wanted the prescription just in case, and his response was, "I want to tell you, Doc, that ever since our sex life got back to normal, I don't need the Viagra anymore. I think my years of affairs put an emotional strain on me and that made me need Viagra. Now I'm happy and relaxed, and I don't need it."

I learned so much from this couple. First, sex doesn't end with age. It may even become intensified and reinvigorated. Second, women often struggle though hormonal changes, and if couples don't expect that and accept that they need both to make adjustments and modify their expectations, it can destroy relationships. Third, if women confront these issues bravely, as this lady did when she agreed to see a counselor, they can be overcome. Fourth, ED can be emotionally driven and can be treated successfully without medicine. Finally, sex is a gift that should be enjoyed and cherished for life. Don't give up on it.

MY STORY

WHEN I BEGAN MY JOURNEY into medicine, I did not anticipate that I would be learning so much from my patients. I began life in Baghdad, Iraq, part of a community of about one hundred and fifty thousand Jews living in the ancient city of the Babylon. But political pressures forced us to emigrate from that country, and I ended up happily moving to and living in Israel.

After I completed high school, I was accepted to the Hadassah Medical School at the Hebrew University of Jerusalem and graduated in 1967. As a young physician, I served my obligatory duty in the Israeli army for three years as a medical doctor. During that period, I also served as a country doctor for a population in a remote area of Israel. Thereafter, I moved with my wife and daughter to New Orleans for training in internal medicine and cardiology. In 1974, after my training, we settled with our three children in Clearwater, Florida, I got my license to practice medicine there, and since that time I have been practicing internal medicine and cardiology as a solo practitioner in Clearwater.

It is hard to believe that I could practice medicine for forty-five years, but my wife, Ella, refuses to let me retire. I think she's afraid that if I stopped working, I would just be home and getting in her way. But the real reason is that I have enjoyed my practice and my patients and the work that I do. As medicine has changed, I have witnessed the changes that have taken place in our lives, our society, and our technology. Through it all, I still believe there is no better machine than what God gave to humans.

From the beginning of my practice, I have always spent as much as an hour with each new patient—listening, asking questions, and paying attention to the patient as a whole person. This was not what I was taught in medical school. Most of my colleagues had a routine system of taking basic health information: "Do you have headaches? Do you have palpitations? Do you have heart disease?" They come across as mechanics working on an automobile.

This is the common way among most physicians today. They have switched their attention and priority from the patient to medical record production and data entry. The physician spends more time, energy, and attention on producing the digital record than on communicating with the human being sitting across the table. This creates unhappy patients and unsatisfied physicians, leads to medical errors, and results in frustrated physicians who are forced to practice medicine according to how insurance companies and lawyers dictate.

This is not only a problem in the primary care environment. One interesting study[1] used sensors to determine how much time physicians on an intensive-care ward spent with patients, and the results were not encouraging. Doctors spent only about 14 percent of their time in patient rooms, compared with about 40 percent in the physician workroom. That's not what young people aspire to do when they decide to embark on the challenging road to become physicians. That's administration.

WHAT I LEARNED FROM TIME WITH MY PATIENTS

I LEARNED MY WAY FROM one of my professors. He said, "I will spend one hour with my patient taking his history. I don't want anybody else to do it for me. I will examine them, and I will determine what's wrong with these patients." This was a very busy professor, but he took the time with everyone, and I admired him because he showed me that good medicine is personal. Good medicine is not the doctor sitting there, asking, "Do you have any eye problems?" and typing without even looking at you. Today, it's not even the doctor; that information will be obtained by an assistant clerk working in the medical office.

That certainly wouldn't work with my focus on sexuality. What would I do if someone came to me with a sore throat? Take a five-minute history on the computer, then say, "Open your mouth and say 'Aah,' and by the way, do you have trouble getting an erection?" He would look at me like I was crazy.

I get the same information in my medical history that other physicians do—about cardiac health, gastrointestinal health, and so on. I ask if they have flatulence, diarrhea, constipation, hemorrhoids—everything that may bother them. If it's a woman, how is her bladder function? If it's a man, how is his prostate function? But I do it at my pace, and I make it a conversation, not an interrogation. Finally, I'll ask "You're married more than ten years— how is your marriage? How is your sex life? Do you have a happy marriage? Do you get along with your spouse well?" Depending on the responses, I'll ask more questions about erectile dysfunction, menopause, or whatever is appropriate. But it is always personal, unhurried, and compassionate. This is where trust begins.

Despite the fact that I wasn't sure how people would respond to sexual and intimate questions raised by me during their routine doctor visit, I felt enough confidence to give it a trial run. To my surprise, my sexual inquiries have not only not offended my patients but were *welcomed*. People were hungry and eager to speak with somebody about their intimacy, feeling that it had been hidden in the dark and surrounded by secrecy.

During forty-five years of practicing medicine in this way, I have learned many important lessons that I never found in medical books or heard from my professors or colleagues. I found the connection between sexuality and many important mental and physical disorders and saw that I could help patients enjoy better overall health by addressing their sexual disorders. My method enabled me to gain my patients' trust and encourage them to be open about intimate issues, helping me deliver more effective care.

The turning point that showed me the connection between sexuality, happiness, and health came during my internship rotation into cardiovascular care. I met with a man, forty-two years old, who had suffered a heart attack. I asked him about other health problems, and there was no pattern. It didn't make sense that this young man would have a heart attack—until I found out that three months earlier, he had begun to experience erectile dysfunction, which shocked and deeply scared him. He felt that his life had turned upside down and that its joy was gone.

Some years later, in 1990, a Japanese physician named Sato described the acute connection between severe emotional crisis and heart injury. Called Takotsubo Cardiomyopathy, or "Broken Heart Syndrome," it can actually lead to heart muscle damage in the presence of normal coronary arteries. A sudden, unexpected emotional crisis will transfer stress from the nervous system into the heart muscle, and this neuro-cardiovascular mechanism can and does cause serious damage to the heart.

You've heard about people with plaques in their coronary arteries caused by years of high cholesterol. Eventually, a plaque deposit ruptures, a blood clot forms, circulation is blocked to the heart, and they have a heart attack. But some heart attacks can occur because of *angiospasm*, a spasm in an otherwise healthy coronary artery. The artery is not blocked, but the blood supply to the heart is occluded by the spasm just the same, leading to heart muscle death. Guess what can cause angiospasm? Emotional distress![2]

Also, in a patient with a partially blocked coronary artery who suffers great emotional distress, arterial plaque can be broken off or ruptured by a drastic change in blood pressure, causing a clot, blockage, heart attack, and possibly death. What I speculated was that, strange as it seemed at first, this patient's heart attack had probably come about as a result of stress caused by his extreme emotional reaction to his unexpected sexual dysfunction.

This young man felt lost when he encountered the unexpected failure in his sexual capacity. He perceived that he was facing a sudden catastrophe. He told me that he began to experience heart palpitations when he tried to perform sexually. Sex became a major source of stress, shame, and fear for him, and chronic stress has many negative physiological effects, including high blood pressure and a narrowing of the coronary arteries due to spasm. Eventually, the acute and chronic stress building in him led to a heart attack.

EMOTION MAKES SEXUALITY
A MEDICAL ISSUE

THIS CONNECTION BETWEEN EMOTION and the neuro-psychiatric system, which is carried through the neuroendocrine system to target organs like the heart and intestine, is what led me to focus on the sexuality of my patients in order to understand them and be able to help them.

For many physicians, sexuality is still a blind spot. They still insist that their patients' sex lives have nothing to do with them providing medical care. That is shortsighted and untrue. Sexuality is an important and integral physiological function. Sexuality in humans is attached to powerful emotions, identity, relationships, and self-image, and a crisis in those delicate areas can produce very real physical and mental symptoms that impair health and well-being. That makes sexuality very much part of the physician's sphere of care.

Imagine a male patient who becomes frustrated by his low sex drive or because he is not satisfied due to rejection from his partner. He will feel inferior, upset, and hurt. He will go to bed with this feeling, and his mind will keep wandering all night, and he will suffer from sleep deprivation. As a result of poor sleep, his blood pressure will keep increasing. He will feel tired, exhausted all day, and lose his interest in exercise. He may go to his doctor and ask for blood pressure treatment and complain of chronic fatigue, possible weight gain, depression, and so on, depending on his personality and the depth of his sexual frustration. But if the physician knows about his sexual problems and understands their potential impact on his health, the physician could spare the patient many unnecessary tests, consultations, and medications.

These are two of the key insights that I have picked up about patients and their sexuality:

- **ED is not a disease.** It is a term invented by the pharmaceutical industry after stumbling on Viagra's positive effect on the erection due to the improved function of the autonomous circulatory system—noticed, as often happens, during research for something else, in this case heart drugs. By the way, this drug was found to increase the blood flow to the woman's vaginal circulatory system, as well.

  A man experiencing ED (what we used to call impotence) will feel emasculated and stripped of his manhood and identity and will believe himself to be a failure. Worse, without treatment, the fear and shame of this problem will perpetuate in all his sexual encounters after the first accidental episode, leading to a chronic inability to perform. Without help, the emotional effects of ED can start a downward spiral that leaves a man questioning his self-worth and destroys his self-esteem. Given that about half of men over age forty are experiencing this condition in various ways, ED qualifies as a crisis. Or as a 2008 study published in the *Journal of Sexual Medicine* concluded, "Erectile function and the effect of ED on aspects of the sexual experience emerged as the most pressing concerns among male participants."[3]

- **Low libido is as traumatic for women as ED is for men; however, it is directed onto a different path.** Low libido, or low sex drive, is most common in women, and it's even less understood than ED. Even if we give a woman after menopause hormonal treatment with added testosterone, that may not rejuvenate her libido.

Here is what I commonly see: after the birth of her child or after she begins menopause, a woman will find that she has little or no interest in sex. Shocked and confused, she will hide her lack of interest from her husband and play the "too tired to have sex" game. The man wants sex, but the woman doesn't care about it. If this is not addressed, the outcome can be devastating: conflict, marital problems, behavioral changes, infidelity, and divorce.

Later, I will talk at much greater length about ED, low libido, their catastrophic emotional and psychological effects, and the different ways that men and women experience sexuality. For now, it's enough to point out that the more I learned, the more I began to build my medical career around practices that helped me build the trust that would gain me admittance to the most private areas of my patients' lives.

Through my patients' intimacy, I learned more about the connection of sex to many other medical disorders, symptoms, and behaviors. This opened the door to understanding and identifying better with my patients. Trust grew, which was not only important for treating conditions that have a strong psychological component, but just as important in treating any medical condition because we are all one unit—the physical and emotional working together. Most patients saw my approach as unique and beneficial and came back to see me again.

WOMEN SHOULD NOT SURRENDER
TO MENOPAUSAL SYMPTOMS

A man was sixty-eight years old, and his wife was sixty-two. They used to have good sex until six years earlier. Thereafter, the wife declined her husband's attempts to start sexual activity and never discussed it with anybody, including her gynecologist. Sex had become painful due to vaginal dryness, and she didn't want to endure the pain. But she never spoke to her husband about this.

The husband grew impatient, not able to understand the reason. He gave up on his wife and started an affair with his neighbor, a married woman who responded to him during the periods when her husband was traveling due to his job. The wife found out about the affair, became furious, and demanded a divorce. This man loved his wife but couldn't reconcile his love with his need for sex.

Both were my patients, and I knew most of the story. When the wife finally admitted to me that she loved her husband but didn't want to have sex because of the pain, it was clear that this husband and wife were victims of secrecy and lack of communication. I convinced her to use estrogen vaginal cream and lubricating jelly, and I encouraged her to give her husband another chance. I also asked them to resume sexual activity. Quickly, their marriage was revived, and they returned to their previous, happy life. Ironically, the neighboring couple (who had both been having affairs) ended up divorcing.

This was a happy ending, but the crisis could have been avoided if the woman had been open to talking about her symptoms and had not assumed that not having sex was okay with her husband.

HOW I RUN MY OFFICE

IN MORE THAN A HALF-CENTURY of involvement in medicine, I have seen a disturbing trend: patients running from specialist to specialist, being tested and treated for depression, irritable bowel and stomach pain, headaches, heart palpitations, and so on. They submit to tests and screenings that find nothing. They take unnecessary medications that sometimes in themselves can cause symptoms and side effects (including, in some cases, ED and loss of libido). They waste time and money, experience false positive or false negative results that can lead to more tests and stress, and get nowhere.

While I was building my practice and asking my patients about their sex lives, I started to realize that sex was the missing link between these people and their inexplicable diseases and disorders. In my experience, about 30 percent of my patients have disorders that turn out to be related to unaddressed sexual problems and the psychological stress that accompanies them, including:

- chest pain
- palpitations
- hypertension
- type 2 diabetes
- depression
- anxiety
- headaches
- GI symptoms
- insomnia
- weight gain
- poor diet

- low motivation
- chronic pain
- rashes and other skin problems
- immune disorders
- addiction and impulse control[4]

Those are just some of the physical and mental symptoms that research shows can result from the kind of unrelenting stress that men and women often feel when their sex lives are in turmoil. There are a lot of others. Some of this is explained by a relatively new science called psychoneuroimmunology, which studies the relation between mental states, nervous system function, and the immune system. Chronic stress floods your body with hormones like cortisol and adrenaline, and over time these can alter how your brain functions[5], impair your immune system's ability to fight disease[6], interfere with your endocrine system's ability to regulate your blood sugar[7], and a lot more.

Those are just the direct effects of sexual stress. There are other effects of poor sex lives (also supported by research) that doctors don't take into account but should. I call these "quality of life outcomes," and I have seen them over and over again in my practice:

- higher divorce rate
- higher infidelity rate
- lower marriage satisfaction
- lower confidence
- impaired body image and body dysmorphia
- irritability
- sleep disorders
- loss of interest in sex

- taking unnecessary medication or undergoing unnecessary treatment
- negative effects on children's development

These quality of life factors have at least as great an impact on patients' happiness as their weight, cholesterol level, or blood sugar—and truthfully, they are much more important in determining whether a patient is content or miserable. But over the years I have found few physicians in any specialty who treat ED, low libido, or lack of transparency about sex as real health problems that deserve their attention. That is why I determined to run my medical practice according to a different set of priorities, despite the financial losses that come with spending lots of unreimbursed time with patients talking about their sex lives.

For one thing, I never have anyone else in the room when I am speaking with or examining a patient. That privacy creates a sense of intimacy and helps the patient get past any sense of being judged for what he or she says. This one-to-one time helps foster the idea that we are collaborating on the patient's health.

I conduct what is probably one of the most thorough patient histories in medicine, including questions about the state of their marriage, sexual relations, frequency of sex, orgasm, and so on. Every patient I have seen has been open, even eager, to talking about these topics, and many of them express satisfaction and remark that no other doctor they have ever seen has asked them such questions and given them such a thorough examination, though they wish they had. In the beginning, I was surprised to find that patients welcomed my questions, but then I came to understand that they were all victims of the current state of medicine—made to feel that the only thing that mattered was their symptoms, not who they were and how they felt as human beings.

I also listen closely and respectfully to my patients, writing down information by hand, not on a computer or tablet. This lets me pay close attention to what they say, how they say it, and their body language. This is all a part of building trust while studying the patient. Many of these people may never have spoken about their secret sexual fears or shame to anyone. That is a crippling burden to bear. By asking patients about their sex lives and their marriages and treating the answers as important and consequential, I learn about the real person presenting the symptoms and I gain their confidence. Through that process they become more likely to follow my medical instructions and benefit from treatment.

Patients come not only to hear what you have to say as a doctor but also for you to listen to them, too!

THE HEALING POWER OF TRUST

I THINK ONE OF THE REASONS I have seen such amazing results in people's mental and physical health once they take my advice about sexual difficulties in their lives is because of the power of trust. When a patient trusts me, he or she will follow my instructions to the letter. You have heard of the placebo effect, in which the belief that a treatment will be effective often produces the same—or better—results than actual treatment. The placebo effect exists in every treatment and in every pill and often has an important role in curing the disease. I once wondered why one patient with pneumonia will recover while the other one will not when both are given the same medicine. But my observations frequently showed that the one who recovered possessed higher confidence in the treatment than the other one. If we as physicians promote patients' trust and faith in what we are doing for them in addition to effective medical treatment, we can achieve double the benefit for them.

What do I mean by this? I mean that on many occasions, my male patients have been cured of ED simply by me finding out and telling them that there was nothing physically wrong with them or by them talking openly with their wives about their fears. No Viagra. Nothing but confidence. That is the power of the placebo effect. Science has shown us that when patients simply believe they have received an effective treatment, they will often have a positive physiological response. We see that in medical research when we try a new medication and compare it to the placebo in blind tests and find that about 30 percent of patients given the placebo experience the same effect as the subjects who took the medication. Studies have shown that even patients given a placebo after surgery experienced the same pain relief as patients who had taken actual analgesics . . . as long as they *believed* the placebo was a painkiller.[8] That is the power of the mind.

As a physician, I have far more power to heal my patients—or to help them heal themselves—when they trust that I care about them and have their best interests at heart, and that what I am telling them to do will really help them. That's what has been lost in medical care today with the way so many doctors are forced to practice. They are overwhelmed with computer work, paperwork, and bureaucracy, stressed by the legal and financial system and the excessive number of patients that they have to see, and often crushed by medical school debt. Consequently, physicians are burned out, unhappy, and depressed. They can't enjoy the career they have worked so hard for. And without motivated physicians willing to commit to their patients, patients become victims, feeling that they have nowhere to turn for help.

Happiness and depression are contagious. When physicians are unhappy with their work, patients can "catch" their misery and become even more unwell. Instead, let us infect our patients with joy and happiness—let us do in medicine what makes us happy.

The Toll Modern Medicine Takes on Doctors

Medicine used to be one of the careers that everyone aspired to. Now the modern health-care industry is forcing physicians to work so long and hard that they are suffering. Reform is critical for both doctors and their patients. For example:

According to the "Medscape National Physician Burnout & Depression Report 2018," 42 percent of the fifteen thousand physicians surveyed said they had experienced burnout, and another 15 percent felt some level of depression.

The number one reason for burnout? Too many bureaucratic tasks.

According to a 2014 review published in the Medical Student Research Journal, *physicians are more likely to abuse prescription drugs than the general population. And a 2013 study by the University of Florida reported that 10 to 15 percent of doctors surveyed had developed a substance-use disorder.*

Physicians have the highest suicide rate of any professional, ranging from twenty-eight to forty suicides for every one hundred thousand people. The overall rate in the general population is 12.3 per one hundred thousand.[9] I find it ironic that physicians who were trained to save lives cannot save their own lives. Personally, I save the pain pills for rainy days when I have pain.

CHANGING THE FUTURE

THE WAY I PRACTICE MEDICINE is still the exception, not the rule, and that is part of the problem. I think it is very important not only for physicians to speak openly and compassionately with patients about their sexual lives or other issues that occupy the patients' minds, but also to be free to operate their practices as they see fit. In this way, they will be able to actually *enjoy* practicing medicine—which, after all, is the reason we all got into this demanding profession.

One thing the government can do is to get lawyers out of the business of influencing medical decisions. Leave patient care in the hands of the physician. Cover every patient with basic medical care and offer the wealthy access to private medicine if they want the extra care. Stop forcing doctors to rely on insurance company bureaucracies to get compensation and allow things to run simply and efficiently by eliminating the corporate profit incentive. This will result in better care, which in turn will save everyone money.

We must also intervene to reduce the influence of the pharmaceutical industry on what doctors say and do. There are medications that work miracles and save lives, certainly; I have seen Viagra alone save marriages and radically change the condition of people's marriages and save some men from mental agony.

But this goes beyond regulation or laws. Why is medicine ignoring such a fundamental, essential part of the human experience as sexuality? I will dig into this more deeply later in the book, but for now I will say that I believe that corporate medicine has made many doctors forget about the healing power of empathy, trust, and listening. We overlook it because handing someone a pill and entering data into a database gets us paid.

Research shows that empathy on the part of the physician does not just make the patient feel better but actually contributes to the physiological act of healing.[10] That is extraordinary. But I believe the effect of empathy and trust goes even further than its impact on the brain. Our society is flooded with anxiety from the news, social media, and more. Anxiety is a plague of our time, and it is one of the chief causes of many of the physical symptoms I've talked about in this chapter. Anxiety has penetrated our homes and daily lives; it is contagious and poisonous. But one of the most powerful tools we have to deal with and let go of that anxiety— healthy, loving, communicative, pleasurable sex with our loved one—is being neglected because physicians and patients won't talk about the problem!

We act like cattle, led by social taboo, labeling sex as sinful and dirty. Unsure, laypeople stay silent, even husbands and wives. Uncomfortable, physicians stay silent, as well, unwilling to deal with the taboo and preferring to stay on the mechanistic side of medicine. And with that silence comes ignorance.

People may think that if they have a sexual problem, something is wrong with them, when in reality it may be a false assumption or just a normal age-related issue. But they won't ever know if they or their doctor won't talk about it! Others make the awful mistake of accepting that if their sex life is bad today, there is no hope or remedy. They will either have to live with a sexless marriage for the rest of their lives or leave their marriage and destroy their family. But nothing could be further from the truth. Great sex is not only possible but probable into our seventies, eighties, and beyond . . . but only if we break the silence and understand that almost every sexual dysfunction can be treated in some way or other.

Interestingly, when patients have back pain, stomach cramps, or ringing in the ears, they will never say, "I need to live with it," or "I am not normal because of this problem." They will go to doctors to find out how to fix it. But for sexual problems, too many people accept them, hide them, and suffer in silence.

Almost every situation in which one or both partners are not achieving sexual satisfaction can be solved with communication, patience, openness, and love.

In other words, *there is always hope.*

Sexual problems in our society are more common than depression, irritable bowel syndrome, or even arthritis. But they have been concealed in the silence of myth and taboo. It is time for the epidemic of silence about sexuality to end. Time for physicians to engage with their patients and take back their profession. Time to get past the taboos and talk about sexuality candidly and without judgment. Time to respect sex as what it is: a vital part of a complete life, a happy marriage, and lifelong wellness.

Time to recognize that sex is not an animal act and can be discussed in the open without shame or fear.

Chapter Three

TWO DIFFERENT MACHINES

F or years, there has been a joke making its way around the internet that illustrates the difference between men and women. It takes the form of diary entries, one from a wife and the other from her husband:

Wife's Diary:

Tonight, I thought my husband was acting weird. We had made plans to meet at a nice restaurant for dinner. I was shopping with my friends all day long, so I thought he was upset at the fact that I was a bit late, but he made no comment on it. Conversation wasn't flowing, so I suggested that we go somewhere quiet so we could talk. He agreed, but he didn't say much. I asked him what was wrong. He said "nothing." I asked him if it was my fault that he was upset. He said he wasn't upset, that it had nothing to do with me, and not to worry about it. On the way home, I told him that I loved him. He smiled slightly and kept driving. I can't explain his behavior. I don't know why he didn't say, "I love you, too." When we got home, I felt as if I had lost him completely, as if he wanted nothing to do with me anymore. He just sat there quietly and watched TV. He continued to seem distant and absent. Finally, with silence all around us, I decided to go to bed. About fifteen minutes later, he came to bed. But I still felt that he was distracted and his thoughts were somewhere else. He fell asleep. I cried. I don't know what to do. I'm almost sure that his thoughts are with someone else. My life is a disaster.

Husband's Diary:
Motorcycle won't start . . . can't figure out why.

That's funny, but the differences between men and women are very real, and that is no truer than when we talk about sexuality and sexual gratification. One of the chief causes of friction and conflict in marriages is the fact that men and women derive pleasure from sex in different ways. Of course, the idea that sex exists not only for reproduction but for pleasure, as well, is a fairly recent notion and remains radical to some people. However, not in my tradition, the Jewish tradition.

In the Torah, the source of the Bible, Moses says in an oration to his people, "I have put before you life and death, blessing and curse. Choose life, that you and your descendants may live!" In this context, "life" means pleasure and joy as well as making new generations of Israelites. Man is the only creature for whom sex is a source of enjoyment, intimacy, bonding, and freedom, as well as a means to reproduce. Sexual sharing affects the health of the individual, the marital union, and the family.

The Hebrew Talmud was written by rabbinical scholars after the destruction of the second temple, and they dedicated much of the book to the interrelations between husband and wife. As much as one would think that those scholars had nothing to do with sex, amazingly, they described in detail how the man and the woman should act sexually to each other, even when God is watching them. They wrote guidance for almost every question that might ever come up in such situations. This could be one of the reasons that Jewish families have been so strong over the generations, with less divorce and more united families.

So how is it possible that we have omitted this knowledge from our health system and society? How have we remained so ignorant about the differences between men and women? Sex can be a powerful force for good in our lives if we choose to channel it that way. Healthy sexuality only benefits the marriage and family and, in doing so, benefits all of society. When men and women are more intimate and loving, they treat each other with more compassion and respect. They show their children more love and care and model an example of a healthy family. Those qualities are passed along to generations in the future. Sex is a force for positive change.

However, if we deny the sexual appetite—or, as so many religions have done, turn it into something forbidden, a sin and a shame—we twist the sexual impulse into a source of evil. Sexual frustration, including the inability to resolve ED, is at the core of much of the rage, violence, and impulse to sexually assault that we see in men, who behave as wild animals. Self-loathing over lack of sexual desire is a chief cause of depression, self-hatred, and even suicidal thinking in women.

It is time to correct this problem. It has been sitting on our doorstep for generations awaiting attention, and we must address it respectfully. Let us do so.

MEN AND WOMEN ARE NOT THE SAME

HOW DO WE CHOOSE the good in sex? We begin by understanding that men and women are *not* the same when it comes to sexual function or sexual pleasure. We are two different machines that work in two different ways on different fuels, testosterone versus estrogen. Only when we acknowledge and accept that can we successfully operate these two machines as a single, strong, powerful, and efficient unit. We can complement one another sexually, which means that we have talked to each other and learned about the other partner's sexuality as much as our own. This means taking the time to learn about our sexuality in the same way that we learn about our blood pressure, cholesterol, kidney function, blood sugar levels, and other basic aspects of our health and attaching as much importance to our sexual function as we do to those other areas.

This patient story illustrates what can happen when we don't acknowledge these differences, something that usually happens due to ignorance. I saw a woman, fifty years old, with a husband, fifty-one and healthy. They have three children. But in our conversation, she told me that her husband was frustrated. He was focusing on his successful career, working late, and they hadn't had sex in five years.

Imagine if I hadn't asked about their sex life! They hadn't talked about it with each other, so how would anything ever be solved without me asking? A life with no sex became their normal life. They just accepted it and were miserable, living in the darkness with each other's secrecy.

But life is a gift. You have the gift. You should use it and enjoy it. I pressed the woman to talk further, and she told me that her husband had given up on her because he said he was fatigued and aching all the time. These were excuses. She told me that she knew that he loved his family and he would never have an affair. So he masturbated to satisfy his sexual needs; however, he was unhappy doing it, which he acknowledged to me. She also knew that he still found her attractive and sexy because of comments he made and the way he looked at her. So what was the problem? The situation sounded strange to me: on one hand, the man had a sexual urge and his wife was there and willing, so why would he choose to satisfy himself by masturbation instead?

I asked more questions and found out that after she had given birth to their last child, she had experienced chronic nonspecific symptoms like fatigue, depression, poor concentration, and more. But the most devastating symptom was that she had lost her libido, her interest in sex. She did nothing about it but felt shame over this and used excuses to turn her husband's advances down. Finally, frustrated, he gave up on her and satisfied his drive by masturbation. That pulled them apart from each other. She never talked to her husband about her problems but kept them to herself.

During this long period of sexual separation, something built up in both of them. The woman lost a sense of her femininity and satisfaction in being a woman who was attractive and wanted because she thought that her husband was not interested in her sexually. On the other hand, the man felt that she was no longer attracted to him sexually. That made him withdraw from her out of injury to his pride and dignity and abandon sexual relations with the woman he loved. They were both losers, and neither of them talked about it.

Feeling lost and rejected, she converted her unhappiness to symptoms—to disease. She went from doctor to doctor, specialist to specialist, wondering what was wrong with her. Not one of them could identify a specific disease or give her a specific diagnosis. Basically, she was a healthy woman. So, unable to find any physical cause for her symptoms, she started to put the blame on her husband.

She accused him of not communicating and not caring about her. In her mind, he gave up on her. His only interest was his work, and he had no time to spend with her. He got sex through masturbation and didn't even approach her anymore. She told me that she didn't even feel that she knew him anymore, and that she was beginning to wish she had never met him. They were very close to the destruction of their marriage. She was thinking about divorce when I saw her.

After she poured out all her pain to me, I asked her, "Where would you go if you got divorced? Do you expect better relations with another man?" Then I asked her why she had given her husband the cold shoulder for so long when it came to sex. She told me she hadn't even thought about that and never associated sex with their relationship issues.

"I wake up in the morning. Every day I don't feel the drive. What am I supposed to do?" she asked. That was the heart of the problem, I told her. Loss of sex drive is very common for women as they age, but most women don't know that. So, in dealing with that loss and the feelings of guilt and rejection that come with it, they just rely on their instinct. Some women have the right instinct, but many others have the wrong instinct in how to respond to the loss of libido.

What is the wrong instinct? It's doing nothing. It's saying, "I'm not thirsty, I'm not going to drink water." It's feeling tired and sitting on the couch instead of getting up and exercising. In other words, many women with low libido don't understand the importance of sex in their marriage and its effect on their life, so they assume that they can just end sexual relations altogether and it will somehow be all right with their self-image, their husbands, and their relationship. They fail to understand that for most men, the sex drive remains strong throughout his life. He not only wants sex but *needs* it.

I told her about this, but I did not place all the blame on her. "Your husband also has responsibility here because he did not talk to you about your lack of interest in sex," I said. "He simply tuned you out because of resentment and focused on his work and on taking care of himself through masturbation." I said that in my opinion, her husband was not a bad man who didn't love her but instead, like many other men, was ignorant of the changes in libido that affect many women. He assumed that she was *choosing* not to want sex, when in reality the biological need was just not there. Again, ignorance led to silence, resentment, blame, and anger.

But the wife was my patient, and she was a good woman who was struggling with many somatic symptoms. I thought I could help her solve this problem with some honest discussion, so I got to the issue. I explained in detail the difference between the male and female libido that often comes along when both are in their fifties, which is when I usually see it. I said, "Your husband needs sex biologically. That does not make him a sex maniac; it makes him a healthy man." I explained that her low libido was also very common. Then I told her, "If your husband is hungry, you cannot give him a book to read. You have to give him food." I asked her to talk with him about their problems and their misunderstandings and to start sexual activity with him even if she did not feel the desire. She was receptive to these ideas and said she would try for the purpose of reigniting her own sexual energy, motivation, and drive on the one hand, and for rebuilding her marriage and family unity on the other.

Six months later, I saw the woman again. She told me that she had taken my advice and, in doing so, had become closer than ever with her husband. They are having sex, and he no longer feels deprived. Things were much better between them. She was still struggling with her libido, although it had significantly improved, and while she was not usually reaching orgasm, she was enjoying the other benefits of sexual activity, such as intimacy, being loved and wanted, feeling attractive to her husband, and being able to satisfy him sexually. They were a happier couple, and she was a happier woman. They have not divorced, and their marriage is getting stronger.

And all the symptoms she had seen all those doctors for? They are gone.

The appalling part of this otherwise hopeful story is that I am the only person, doctor or otherwise, who ever talked with this woman about her sexuality, her libido, and how sexlessness would affect her marriage and her health. *That* is the problem.

HOW THE TWO MACHINES WORK

THE REMEDY BEGINS WHEN WE start to get past judging each other for our sexuality and understanding a very, very basic reality about men and women:

They are not the same sexually in any way,
and there is nothing wrong with that.

We need to accept and understand this fact of nature and learn its rules and fundamentals. The more we know of it, the better we will understand how to use and benefit from it. The basic problem is that we believe we know about our own sexuality and that you should make the effort to learn everything you can about it. However, many people do not know or fully understand their own sexuality. Just assume you are ignorant because that will place you in a position to inquire and learn about it. The best way to do that is also to talk to your partner and ask questions. The ultimate way to know each other sexuality is to openly and bravely talk to each other.

Men and women have different sexual needs and sex drives, and they get sexual satisfaction in different ways. But in order to fulfill their needs, they must work together and understand each other. Do not assume that what works for you sexually will work for your partner, because it probably will not.

In fact, the difference between male and female sexuality could be the single most important factor affecting our marriages and relationships. Because we don't know about the differences or we pretend they don't exist, we end up judging our partners for not responding the way we want them to or expect them to respond using the parameters we apply to ourselves. That leads to both partners not understanding each other because they are each using a different language with its own code. Remember the tower of Babel? When God decided to destroy their ability to build the tower, he simply made it so that everyone spoke a different language. That created chaos, ending in the tower's collapse.

Men and women need a common language they can use to understand each other's sexuality and communicate clearly about issues and challenges. This begins by understanding how both sides' sexuality works and accepting that the two are not the same. Take this couple:

He was fifty-two, she was forty-four. They lived together unmarried for eight years and had a child together. When I asked him about sex, he told me that they had not had sex in three years because she would not respond to him. When he asked her why, she would say, "I don't want to talk about it." After a while, he stopped asking and relieved his urge by masturbation. They were both very upset and unhappy with the situation, and they never discussed how they were feeling or what they needed. The secrecy and the distance between them built up. Finally, he concluded that this was not the life he wanted, and he planned to leave her and come to some agreement with her about custody of their child.

This was why the Tower of Babel collapsed: there was no communication, and people brought the disaster on themselves. This couple's situation was a tragedy to me: a single mother raising a child because the parents went their separate ways. But more tragic was that they didn't know the real reason why their relationship was ending. I can attest that I frequently see stories similar to this one, and I expect that if they asked each other the questions I ask, most other physicians would say the same thing. This is an enormous social crisis that affects our families and our nation, but the fact that no one will talk about it keeps us from recognizing its dimensions.

Without communication between man and woman, we can expect that conflict and damage in the relationship will take place, leading to undesirable consequences. This will happen despite the fact that both partners will believe they are right and doing their best according to what little they know about their own sexual system.

Therefore, we have to educate ourselves on this topic. Let's begin with the basics: the different biological machinery behind the way that male and female desire, arousal, orgasm, and resolution work. First, the sexual cycle in men:

- **Desire**—Sometimes in response to stimulus (sexual fantasies, the visual stimulus of a pretty girl crossing the street, pornography) and sometimes with no stimulus at all, the areas of the man's brain associated with desire (or libido) become more active. These are the *cerebral cortex* and the *limbic system*. The cerebral cortex is the thinking, planning part of the brain, while the limbic system—which includes areas like the hippocampus and amygdala nucleus—is largely connected to emotion and memory. When a man thinks about sex, these areas begin calling up memories of past sexual encounters and anticipating future sex, sending signals to the nervous system. In turn, this increases blood flow to his genitals, causing an erection. His heart rate and breathing quicken, his skin might become flushed and his nipples erect, and his testicles swell. He is ready for sex.

- **Arousal**—Sex or masturbation is either about to begin or has begun, and the same changes continue. The man's muscles tense, his breathing and pulse continue to accelerate, and his testicles withdraw into his scrotum. He is now completely focused on the sexual act, and his need to reach orgasm may be overwhelming.

- **Orgasm**—After a few minutes (the average man's sexual cycle lasts only about two to seven minutes), blood pressure and heart rate spike, and intense involuntary muscle contractions begin at the base of the penis. The prostate gland releases semen, which mixes with the sperm produced by the testicles, and is forcefully ejaculated from the end of the penis in a powerful release of sexual tension.

- **Resolution**—The changes from the first three phases reverse themselves: blood flow and heart rate return to normal, the skin flush disappears, muscles relax, and fatigue sets in. The endocrine system releases the hormone oxytocin, which stimulates feelings of bonding and intimacy. What's notable about men is that most can only experience a single orgasm at a time, followed by a refractory period ranging from several minutes to several hours, during which the man will not experience libido or regain his erection.

It is worth noting here that what stimulates the man's libido can be very different from what stimulates a woman's libido. Men rarely need emotional intimacy to feel sexual desire, and for some men, emotional intimacy is even a turnoff. Men are more often stimulated by sexual content in media, the sight of someone they find sexually attractive, dirty talk in bed, or memories of past sexual encounters.

Women, as it will become clear, are very different. Here is the female sexual cycle:

- **Desire**—The action in the brain is largely the same for the woman as for the man: the cerebral cortex thinks about sex while other parts of the brain call up memories of past sexual activity and the associated emotions. But what sparks this brain activity is unique to women. Women's libido tends to be more stimulated by emotional intimacy than by overt sexuality: cuddling, intimate conversation, emotional closeness, and sharing. Women can of course also be stimulated by the sight of someone they find sexually attractive or the memory of a past sexual encounter, but they are far more likely than men to want sex because of emotional intimacy. When that occurs, physical changes occur. Genital circulation increases, the woman's clitoris and labia swell, breathing and pulse accelerate, the vagina begins to produce lubricating fluid, the breasts and vaginal walls begin to swell, and the skin may flush.

- **Arousal**—Sex or masturbation begins, and the same changes continue. Respiration and heart rate climb, the muscles grow tense, the vagina continues to swell while its walls grow darker in color, and the woman's clitoris becomes extremely sensitive. It also withdraws under the clitoral hood, which can prevent it from coming into direct contact with the penis (more on that in a moment).

- **Orgasm**—This is an area where women differ strongly from men. Because the clitoris withdraws from direct stimulation by the penis, many women rarely or never reach orgasm through intercourse. For those who do, the process also involves rapidly increasing blood pressure and breathing, followed by a rapid release of muscle tension. Women do not ejaculate like men, and they can also experience multiple orgasms during a single sexual encounter, including orgasms that continue long after the man has withdrawn his penis from the vagina.

- **Resolution**—As with men, this stage involves muscle relaxation, fatigue, and the release of oxytocin, which stimulates feelings of well-being, intimacy, bonding, and closeness. Women do not need a refractory period and can feel sexual desire almost immediately after orgasm. However, according to the work of one Harvard researcher, 75 percent of women do not always reach orgasm through intercourse alone,[1] while according to a 2017 study from *The Journal of Sex and Marital Therapy*[2] only 18.4 percent of women reported that intercourse alone was enough to bring them to orgasm. Men should be prepared to continue stimulating the woman orally or manually if she wants to reach climax.

As you can see, the cycle of sexual activity is extremely complex—one of the most complex systems in the human body, requiring the coordinated action of multiple systems from the brain and nervous system, the endocrine system, the circulatory system, the muscles, and so on. And as with any sensitive system with many moving parts, it is easily disrupted. This is because for women and men, sexuality is as much psychological as it is physiological. Yes, the various physiological systems need to work together in harmony to make sex happen, but the psychological component can either enhance the sexual experience or prevent it from happening, sometimes with catastrophic consequences.

It's this psychology and the nature of what brings men and women sexual pleasure that is at the heart of the problems I am addressing in this book.

Factors That Affect Libido

Libido, the desire for sex, can be increased or dampened by a wide range of factors:

Sexual thoughts—It should not be surprising that thinking and fantasizing about sex makes you want sex.

Exercise—All forms of exercise are good for your libido. They increase energy, improve body image, and reduce stress. But strength training like lifting weights is especially good for increasing sexual desire.[3]

Stress—Chronic stress can upset the body's normal hormone levels and also restrict blood flow, making it more difficult to become aroused.

Poor sleep—Conditions like sleep apnea or simply staying up too late and watching screens can disrupt your sleep and leave you too tired for sex.

Depression—Clinical depression changes how the brain works and can interfere with the processes that lead to sexual stimulation. Some depression medications can also change hormone levels, which in turn can impair libido, while others can enhance libido.

Substance use—A little alcohol can reduce inhibitions, which can be great for sexuality. But too much acts as a depressant on the central nervous system, shutting down sexual arousal. Other anxiety drugs like benzodiazepines (such as Xanax) can also suppress libido. Even marijuana can impair sex because it suppresses the pituitary gland, which regulates testosterone levels.

Medication—Prescription drugs, including beta-blockers and other blood pressure meds, can impair libido and lead to ED in men.

Negative emotions—Poor body image, conflict, feelings of insecurity or fear—these can severely reduce libido, most often in women but also in men.

ED—Men who worry about their sexual performance or fear the humiliation of being unable to get an erection may find themselves withdrawing from sex.

Hormonal changes—Testosterone drives sexual desire in women as well as men, and low levels can impair libido. Increased estrogen levels in women can have the same effect.

WHAT BRINGS MEN AND WOMEN PLEASURE

SEXUALITY IS MUCH MORE COMPLEX than we have been willing to acknowledge, and that is part of the problem. We believe that it is simple, so any problems can be solved simply. But that is not the case. So many factors affect sexual function, sexual desire, and sexual pleasure that we are just beginning to understand some of them while many of them are still a mystery.

For example, exercise. I counsel many of my patients to exercise regularly not only as a way to improve their general health and the cardiovascular system but to improve sexual desire and performance. Exercise is like turning on the engine of a car. Once the engine is on, you will be able to operate other systems: the lights, horn, radio, and so on. Those systems work only when the engine is working, so if you want to cool yourself on a hot day, you don't have to go back home. You just turn the engine on and let the air conditioning do the work.

It is the same with sexuality and exercise. Exercise works the body and burns calories. It sends more oxygen to the brain and the cells. Additionally, it will improve weight and cholesterol. During exercise, the metabolism accelerates and burns glucose and fat as well as the accumulated toxins normally produced during regular metabolism. Those toxins, when they accumulate, can create many undesirable symptoms that we often see in liver and kidney failure.

Exercise has so many benefits that it should be a priority for everyone. We get the instant good feeling that comes from endorphin release while we are burning natural toxins to free the body from depression and the factors that inhibit sexual desire.

Exercise is also important to improve how the body functions.

If you do thirty minutes on the treadmill, you have created a new metabolic reaction in every cell. During exercise, the body will burn calories. But most people don't know that during the following twenty-four hours, the body needs to recover from the cellular changes that happen during exercise, and this repairing process requires even more energy. It is like someone investing money: when the investment matures, he will receive the principal payment plus interest. With exercise, the calories burned during activity and during recovery help keep us trim and strong.

The point is, the body wants to be active. It's an active, dynamic system that needs to move, just like an airplane must keep moving forward to stay in the air. We will not remain functioning and healthy by just sitting on the couch. When a woman with low libido comes to me, I give her homework that includes forty-five minutes of exercise per day. Nearly every time, she comes back and tells me, "I'm doing much better now. We're enjoying our sex more." Things turn positive. Why? Because when you operate the engine of the body, everything works better.

I treated a couple—a woman, forty-six years old with a husband, forty-eight years old—who were having no sexual activity due to poor libido. They had both gained weight over the previous six years, fifty pounds and forty-five pounds, respectively. No sex, no exercise, and no physical activity, and sex was out because they felt fat and ugly. All they did together was cook and eat. They were both depressed, feeling hopeless, and visiting many physicians to address multiple symptoms. They suffered from poor sleep and were on various medicines.

As I was the only doctor who was interested in their personal and intimate life, they were very receptive to what I had to say. Following a long discussion and listening, I offered them a program:

exercise daily for one hour, start to count calories, and initiate any form of sexual activity at least once a week. The woman was excited to learn they were both healthy and that there was hope they could pull themselves out of the dark tunnel they were in. Their mood changed almost instantly, and they left the office with pride and hope. I noticed the spark of excitement!

It was rewarding to see them six months later. The women had lost twenty-five pounds, and the man had lost thirty pounds. My God, what the mind can do! They exercised daily, engaged in hobbies together, slept well, weren't taking any medications, and had sex one or two times a week. Her libido was much better, and although she reached orgasm only sometimes, she was happy with that. The man wanted to lose more weight so he would not need to use Viagra.

This couple would have remained miserable, wasting their lives and spending money on unnecessary medical care for years, had I not asked about their intimacy. I have learned from my patients that the power of sex as a motivator and energy producer to ignite the mind and the body is without peer. We should never let it go to waste!

However, the most critical misunderstanding we have about sex is related to the differences between how the man and woman get pleasure from sex.

> *Men and women derive pleasure from sex in different ways. Men's pleasure comes almost exclusively from orgasm. While women also enjoy orgasm, women get much of their sexual pleasure from feeling desired, experiencing emotional intimacy with their partner, and satisfying their partner sexually. Reaching orgasm is not the essential requirement of their satisfaction.*

Our failure to understand and accept this reality is the barrier between most couples and happier, healthier relationships. Why? Because when we refuse to see that our partner does not get pleasure from the same things that we do, we put pressure on ourselves to satisfy them in ways that might not be possible or that they might not be receptive to. For example, a man who becomes obsessed with bringing his wife to orgasm through intercourse when she might not be able to climax in that way might come to feel emasculated, leading to psychological ED due to loss of confidence and pride.

What about a woman who hates that her husband always needs to reach orgasm during sex? She might consider him to be a sex fiend who doesn't care about her pleasure when he is in fact just being a typical, healthy male. What if a man thinks that his wife should become aroused in the same way and at the same speed that he does? He might refuse to engage in the kind of foreplay and emotionally intimate behavior that many women need in order to become fully aroused. If she's not interested in the same quick, impersonal sex that he desires, he might get angry with her when in fact he's really the problem. That is how ignorance leads to pain and stress.

Only by fully acknowledging these differences, understanding that they are normal, and adapting to the needs and expectations of our individual partners can we move past the devastation of broken relationships and the many health problems caused by the stress of sexual conflict.

MEN AREN'T AS SIMPLE AS THEY SEEM

WE JOKE A GREAT DEAL about men and sex in our culture. Men are simple sexually, we say; they always want sex and will do anything for it. You can lead a man around by his penis, or you can say, "that man has a big head and a small head." The big one is in his penis, supposedly. But this does a disservice to men because men's sexuality is actually much more complex, both physiologically and psychologically.

For example, I saw a male patient, forty-two, handsome, and married with two children. He was depressed and unhappy. He was having physical symptoms like insomnia and acid reflux. After I asked the usual questions, I asked him about his sex life. He said, "I'm avoiding it." I asked him about it further, and he said, "I have concern. I have fear."

Extensive conversation led him to offer more information. He finally said, "You know, Doc, I don't know how to touch. I'm afraid that I can't do it." He told me that he was afraid when the time came to have sex that he would fail to get or keep an erection and be humiliated. His fear was paralyzing him. This big man appeared to me like a frightened child.

Obviously, he had failed several times in the past, and now he could not overcome his monstrous fear. We talked about sexual function, and the core of the problem became clear. He said, "I think my penis is too small." It turned out that he kept his distance from his wife because, as he said, "I'm afraid she'll somehow discover my defect." This was tragic.

That is the phallus complex, and it's well known in the history of medicine. Many men have an obsession with or anxiety about the size of their penis. Without knowing that, I might have treated his depression and stomach acid and prescribed sleeping pills. But there was more to his problem. He said he believed that with a small penis like his, he couldn't satisfy his wife, even though she had never said anything about being dissatisfied sexually.

I examined him, and everything looked normal. I told him he was healthy and said that in my opinion, his only problem was his fear. His fear had turned his worries about not satisfying his wife into a reality, but not because his penis was small (which, by the way, it was not). I gave him Cialis to build back his confidence, but 70 percent of the therapy was the conversation and my reassurance that he was healthy. After we were done, he said, "I've never talked to anyone about this. I've been afraid to talk about it. It has been sitting in my head since I was a little child."

I knew then that I could change this man's entire future. If I could help him, guide him out of this prison he was in, his life would be completely different. We talked some more, and I told him that it was certain that his wife knew about his "defect" and that it wasn't a defect at all. After we were done, he hugged me and said, "I'm happier. I'm more confident." Then I saw him three months after, and he said he was a different person. He and his wife were having sex two to three times a week, both reaching orgasm, and talking intimately. His physical symptoms were gone. That made my day.

Sex in men is not all about raging desire and an instant erection. Whether we like it or not, most men attach their identity and sense of masculinity to their ability to perform sexually, to their penis size, and to their ability to bring their woman to orgasm. Pornography in particular has brainwashed many men into believing that everything is about having a huge penis. "Big is good, but bigger is better," we're told. But do you know what surveys of women find their preferred penis size is? According to a study, women like a penis that's 6.3 inches long and 4.8 inches in circumference when fully erect. You know how large the average American penis is? About 5.6 inches long and 4.8 inches around when fully erect.[4] So a little bit above average is fine, but a man doesn't need a giant penis to satisfy a woman. In fact, a penis that's too large may make a woman afraid of discomfort or even injury, and those fears are definitely *not* good for sexual desire.

Women differ from one another about the size of penis they prefer. What matters is that a man and woman fit well to each other. There are numerous factors that determine this, and science knows very little about the matter. All I can say is, let nature do the work because it will do it better than anybody else. Let love flourish, and everything will fit well.

Still, the issue of penis size remains an area where men can be very fragile. Let me share with you what happens when men come to see me for a physical. They take off their clothes, but they always leave their underwear on, like little kids afraid someone is watching. I need to ask almost everyone to drop their underwear. I wonder, do they think I have X-ray eyes to check them through their clothes?

Eventually, I have to examine their prostate and genitalia, and when they pull down their underwear, what do you think 95 percent of them do? They shake their penis out of the pubic hair with a bit of embarrassment, like they're waking it up. *Come out and say hello!* They want their penis to be visible and as large as possible, even for me. But I have seen a lot of penises, so nothing is going to impress me. I really don't think that anyone even thinks about this instinctive reaction. I think it's a remnant from a cultural message that *a real man has a large penis.*

The thing is, while male sexuality may seem simple, it is not. Men's sexual function is delicate and more complex than any computer. Several physiological functions need to work in combination at a given time in coordination with the mind and the subconscious. As I've said, the physiological harmony that has to take place for arousal and sex to occur is easily disrupted by something as simple as the fear of premature ejaculation, the fear of failure, or the fear of embarrassment and disappointment. Because of this, problems are not easy to fix—and they become harder to fix if we assume that men are nothing more than sex-starved animals. Here are some of the realities that you may know (or not know):

- Sexual arousal in men is obvious: the man gets an erection.

- Many men believe that without an erection, they cannot satisfy their wives sexually. That is not true, but because so many men assume that only penetration can lead to orgasm (because that's the primary way men reach orgasm), they believe that the inability to have intercourse makes them a failure.

- Male libido is usually quick and might have nothing to do with emotional intimacy. Men can get aroused by attractive women, pornography, memories, fantasies, and even the adrenaline from intense activities that are not sexual, such as adventure sports. A healthy man may have an early morning erection or even subconscious ejaculation.

- For men, sex is a powerful need. This need gives rise to physiological tension that craves release. That release is best accomplished by healthy sexual relations. However, its power can drive some men into irrationality and negative behavior.

- Sex in men represents pride, control, manhood, respect, and independence. This means that losing sexual potency creates an immediate emotional crisis in the man. Women have no clue what their partner goes through after an episode of nonperformance, and how the woman reacts to this can powerfully affect the man's self-esteem.

- For the man, sexual satisfaction is all about orgasm through successful intercourse. If the man does not climax, he feels that sex for him was a failure, and he is unsatisfied.

- Men can achieve self-satisfaction and relief by masturbation, but the man's mind will always fantasize about the female image. When doing this, he may feel shame and guilt because our culture looks at this act in a negative way. Picasso dared to illustrate what man fantasizes about the female body in many of his drawings and sketches. It is incredible to learn what is in the mind of man.

SEX IS A MALE BIOLOGICAL NEED

FOR MEN, SEX IS A physiological and psychological *need*. Men *need* sexual activity to enjoy true well-being. This is not something to be ashamed of; it is how nature made men. Men simply *need* sex, and while that need typically diminishes with age, it exists throughout a man's life. This doesn't mean that a man who wants regular sex from his wife or partner is a pervert or a sex addict. Women do not have the same libido as men do. Sex is a biological need like hunger or thirst. If it is not satisfied, it will lead to

SEXUAL MISCONCEPTIONS DICTATED BY CULTURE

My female patient was sixty-two and raised in eastern Europe. Her husband was American, sixty-eight. They were both retired and had raised three kids. They expected to be having the best time of their lives, but the woman told me that over the past two or three years, her beloved husband had changed. He became short tempered, angry, and unpleasant. When he exploded at her, she would shake and feel depressed. When I asked her about sex, she said that during the past three years, they had no sexual relations because she had vaginal dryness and sex was painful.

She had never talked about sex with her husband, and she just let it go. "I am from eastern Europe," she said, "and we consider sex there just to make children. If you don't like it or it causes pain, you just forget it." She saw no connection between her and her husband's lack of sex and her husband's anger and short temper.

I explained human sexuality to her, especially the male need for sex and the fact that for men, the libido usually remained strong all their lives. I told her that I thought it was likely that her husband's mood swings were due to sexual frustration. She was very receptive, so I prescribed a topical hormone cream for her to treat dryness and instructed her to discuss the problem with her husband and for them both to work on resuming sexual intercourse.

Six months later, she returned to see me, telling me that she was very happy. Her husband's attitude had changed; he had become more calm and pleasant, and they did more things together. Sex was enjoyable, with no more pain, and they engaged in sexual activity one or two times a week. Her husband never had problems with sexual function and was always ready for her advances. With these little changes, life for them both became happy and fun.

frustration, desperation, and irrational behavior. When it remains active, it signals that the man's health is good; when his health is impaired, his sexual systems will be impaired as well.

This is one reason that, in the Talmud, the rabbis concentrated great attention on intimate relations between a man and woman. They described the rules in detail more than fifteen hundred years ago, educating and guiding couples in how to act and ensure their marital union remained strong. Of course, there was a religious aspect to this, but the physical and emotional components were well described. The Talmud served as a guide for the Jewish family over those many years when the Jewish people were scattered all over the world. The rabbis knew that when the sexual bond is strong, the relationship is strong. Perhaps that is why the Jewish family has remained more unified over the generations.

In men, sex is a physical craving driven by testosterone. Yes, testosterone diminishes with age in about 30 percent of men, but even elderly men still have a great deal of it coursing through their veins. For men, sex equals vitality, energy, and ambition. Many men see life and material success as things to be conquered, and they see sex in the same way. That is not abnormal or unhealthy; it is a sign of a man who is virile, vital, and mentally and physically healthy. Sex is also how men express love for women because, in the man's mind, the pleasure of sexual orgasm is the greatest pleasure two people can share. That is why it can be so emotionally devastating for the man when he cannot bring his partner to orgasm.

Still, men can and do experience a loss of libido. If a man's testosterone levels drop too sharply with age, his sex drive may drop as well, and he may experience ED. However, low libido in men can be due to other causes like liver and kidney disease, diabetes, depression, and more. And of course, psychological issues can affect libido, as I've related. If a man fears that he will be humiliated during sex, his desire can dry up. I have had male patients who were ashamed of their sexual appetites as well as their need to masturbate. Women and men should respect the fact that men are more complicated sexually than they might seem.

For example, a male patient of mine was forty-eight years old, his wife, forty-four. They had been married for ten years and had two children. They were a very nice couple, but something seemed to be missing. They led a dull life for a young couple. She took care of the kids, and he worked as an engineer. They got some exercise but mostly stayed home and did not have much of a social life. He was gaining weight but still looked good and healthy. But after I asked, he told me that they seldom engaged in sexual activities. He could perform well, and she had a great desire for sex anytime, so why didn't they have sex?

He told me that he had no libido and no urge for sex. He had never brought it to the attention of anybody, including his wife. After tests were completed, I found that his testosterone was very low. I offered him the hormone, but initially he declined it because of possible side effects; he didn't feel increasing his libido was worth the risk. I explained to him that sex is a gift, and that the higher testosterone levels would give him more drive, motivation, and excitement and the flavor of youth and love. He wasn't convinced until I mentioned that he was accumulating body fat instead of muscle and this would continue, along with the loss of bone mass, as a result of the hormone deficiency. He said he would try the hormone.

I was surprised to see a young man who was not eager for sexual activity but seemed complacent with this. He had never discussed the issue with his wife and never considered her sexual needs. Had he discussed it openly with her and listened to what she had to say, perhaps he would have been motivated to make an effort on her behalf. The hormone treatment was successful in reviving this man's motivation. He started a vigorous exercise program, became involved in social activities, and engaged in various projects. He and his wife renewed their sexual relations, bringing them closer to each other. Their family life became more rewarding and exciting.

> There is a myth that men are sexually attracted only to young women. Yes, there is some truth to this because of evolution. Historically, men have been attracted to younger women with slim waists, clear skin, and large breasts because those were all indicators of fertility. But that does not mean that men are only attracted to younger women. As men age, they find intellect, confidence, wit, and fitness just as attractive. Sexual attractiveness also varies by culture and ethnicity. For example, among the Bushmen of the Kalahari Desert in Africa, the men are attracted to women with big hips. Therefore, the chief of the tribe keeps his women in a cage to avoid exercise and feeds them to enhance the size of their hips.

WOMEN ARE COMPLETELY DIFFERENT FROM MEN

WHEN I SEE WOMEN IN my practice, the story they tell about sex is completely different from the story that men tell. Time and time again, they tell me that the intimacy they receive from sexual relations with their partners gives them most of what they need.

I do not doubt that this is true. In a large survey published in the *Journal of Sex and Marital Therapy*,[5] more than 36 percent of women said they needed clitoral stimulation to reach orgasm, and fewer than 20 percent said that intercourse alone could make them climax. But since men's sexual experience and satisfaction are all about intercourse and orgasm, there must be many women who are not experiencing orgasm at all and yet still enjoying sex. How can this be?

I can answer this question from professional experience. When I ask women about sex without orgasm, they will tell me sincerely, "I got what I wanted. I was satisfied." They are getting satisfaction from emotional and psychological sources: being desired as a woman, emotional and physical intimacy with their partner, and satisfying a man and bringing him to orgasm. Women take great pleasure from this, but men don't know it—and many women think there is something wrong with them if they do not reach orgasm. Others simply resign themselves to never experiencing orgasm because they do not ask their partners to stimulate them in another way or just decide to be happy and satisfied with the other rewards they receive from sex.

I often challenge those women and ask them directly, "If you don't end with orgasm, then why do you want to have sex?" The answer is always something like, "Because it makes me happy to feel wanted and loved and to satisfy my husband." This is why the interaction between man and woman should always work two ways: give and receive. When that woman feels she is only there to satisfy the man, the quality of sex suffers. Therefore, I always stress this point to each partner: give attention and consideration to your partner if you want the same in return.

I had a couple in their early sixties in my office, and I confronted them about their need to understand basic facts. Both of them, while sitting with me, wanted all the facts on the table. They struggled to understand each other and be comfortable in knowing that they were doing the right things to please each other. They felt an imbalance in their sex life that needed explanation and guidance.

I told them that for women, 85 percent of the reward for a sexual encounter will be emotional; the rest will be added by the orgasm. This is not the same for men, whose reward will be almost entirely related to the orgasm. The reward for the woman during sex is mental and emotional—feeling wanted, feeling young, feeling vital, feeling feminine. That emotion doesn't have to come with a big sex drive or a big orgasm. But the husband had a very different concept about his wife's sexual satisfaction. He felt that the man's responsibility is to bring his wife to orgasm. However, this man hadn't been able to bring his wife to orgasm and that was affecting his confidence. By talking about what he didn't know about female desire and pleasure and letting him know how he could please her without orgasm, I took the pressure off him and brought them closer together.

I was able to intervene with that couple, but others are not so lucky. Many women misunderstand their sexuality and assume that if their libido decreases at any age without particular reason or if they cannot reach orgasm through intercourse, they just have to live with it and there is nothing they can do about it. That is untrue. Here are the realities of women's sexual pleasure:

- The female libido is more complex than the male libido and much less understood.

- Loss of libido is the biggest sexual problem affecting women, but it's also poorly understood and seems to be caused by a combination of physiological, social, and psychological factors, including stress, relationship problems, medical issues, medication, and menopause-related hormonal changes. Because of this, low libido in women is rarely "fixed" with a single treatment or single bullet. I have seen loss of libido often in young women after they have given birth. The woman's mind switches to motherhood, and she starts to put all her attention there, making her sexuality an afterthought. When that happens, the outcome can be unfortunate for the family.

Here is one example of what I mean. I had a forty-five-year-old male patient I have known for many years. He was successful in business and devoted to his family and to his wife. They have four children, all healthy and beautiful. One day he visited my office looking sad and depressed. When I asked him to tell me about the problem, he said that he had divorced his wife and was living in an apartment. Shocked, I asked why, and he said, "Doc, I asked for the divorce because I could not take it anymore." He added that he loves his wife and said she is a wonderful mother and a good person.

I said, "Please tell me the reason that you couldn't take it anymore and divorced?" He said that after she gave birth to her last child four years earlier, his wife completely lost interest in engaging in sexual relations. He tried to talk to her, but for some reason she was resigned: no libido meant no sex. After four years of struggling with this life, he decided that the marriage needed to end. This tragedy could have been avoided if I had gotten involved sooner.

- The woman's sexual desire plays a major role in the stability of her family. Because men usually have a strong libido throughout their lives and women do not, the woman ultimately controls the sexual activity in the relationship.

- Sexual arousal is not as obvious in women as in men, but it is made physiologically noticeable by the increase in blood flow resulting in signs like flushing and erect nipples.

- Arousal in women is often linked to emotional intimacy. Many women need foreplay, cuddling, and other precursors to sex before they can feel "in the mood" and have the natural vaginal lubrication that makes sex pleasurable. As women age, it will take longer for arousal to achieve its full effect. For example, a postmenopausal woman who hurries to have intercourse may find it painful because her vagina is slower to produce lubrication.

- For women, more of the pleasure of sex comes from affection, feeling desired, being close, and experiencing physical pleasure than from reaching orgasm. As I have said, only about 20 to 25 percent of women reach orgasm through intercourse alone, but that seems to be much less important to women than it does to men. I have often asked women if they want to continue sexual activity when they know they will not achieve orgasm. They have always answered positively—they enjoy it and it makes them feel desired and closer to their partner.

- Women's ability to reach orgasm, and the type of stimulus that gets them to orgasm (oral, manual, masturbation) varies widely. Unlike men, who follow a predictable sexual cycle and achieve orgasm through an equally predictable set of stimuli, women are less predictable.[6]

The most important fact to know about women is that while female sex is about pleasure and relaxation, it is also about intimacy, sharing, feeling desired, and pleasing their partners. Orgasm, while desirable, is not the be-all, end-all of sex for women. Women rarely exhibit the same primal hunger for sex that men do. It is critically important to understand that *this does not make them frigid or manipulative*. It makes them normal. The man engaging in sex needs to take this under consideration and not assume the woman will have the same expectations that he has. He will find his own pleasure enhanced by being able to satisfy his partner and make her happy.

LOSS OF FEMALE LIBIDO DOESN'T HAVE TO LEAD TO TRAGEDY

RESEARCH HAS SHOWN THAT MEN really do have stronger sex drives than women, and men's sex drives are very direct. When a man becomes aroused, his only goal is to achieve orgasm. Women, on the other hand, are more complex. A woman's libido may depend on feeling understood or supported by her partner. Intensity, passion, and risk tend to stimulate men's libidos, while women tend to crave safety, tenderness, and romance.

These differences are real, but men and women remain shockingly ignorant about them, and that to me is the source of so much of the conflict and pain we see in today's relationships. For example, because many men believe that sex for women is about reaching orgasm in the same way it is for men, they believe that if they fail to bring their partner to orgasm, they have failed as men—they are inadequate. This is not true because women are different. But this causes many problems with men, including psychological ED, which can cause bigger issues such as male loss of libido and the man rejecting the woman's advances.

Another problem comes when men fail to understand that many women do not climax through intercourse. Instead of simply rolling over and going to sleep after orgasm, a man might instead spend time stimulating the woman in other ways. When he learns what gives his particular partner pleasure, he can share with her the same pleasurable release. This not only brings physical pleasure but shows the love and care that are part of female sexual pleasure.

Interestingly, this was also discussed in the Talmud. The rabbis instructed that the man, after achieving his orgasm, should not quit and leave aside his wife in the bed but stay with her to comfort her and share his devotion and loyalty.

I also see problems when men don't understand the female loss of libido, something that is common. Many men come to me frustrated, angry, and ready to end their marriages because they believe their wife is choosing not to have sex and that they don't care about the husband. But most women are not choosing this; the cause is biological and poorly understood and related to the loss of libido. They are not rejecting their husbands! They don't have the urge to engage with sexual activity. If men understood this, they could speak with their wives, see a physician, discuss options, find help, and potentially revive their sex lives and marriages. No couple should end a marriage because of a libido issue; it can almost always be resolved.

This is what I have seen after long years of dealing with this issue. When a woman loses her libido (and it does happen frequently to young women also), it creates serious and unanticipated problems with her relationship, her self-image, and her health. The woman often becomes upset, feeling that she has forever lost something associated with youth and vitality, and often has no idea that there is anything she can do about it. In my experience, few women will search for answers or talk to their physician. They may ask their gynecologist for advice and maybe receive a prescription for hormones. But they will not receive any advice on how to relate to their partners or revive their sexual lives and marriages. This leads to the end of many marriages.

Sadly, so many women bring tragedy to families because of low libido that they are changing the map of our society. Nearly 50 percent of all marriages end in separation or divorce, so increasingly, we have children raised by single mothers who need to work to pay bills, leaving them with no time for themselves or their kids. It saddens me to observe how we got into this problem as a result of such a foolish thing as not understanding the female libido. Of course, that is not the only reason for the high divorce rate or single motherhood, but sexual problems certainly contribute to the destruction of many families.

Many women tend to accept the loss of their libido and never discuss it with anybody. They go silent and become almost asexual. The husband doesn't understand why there is no sex and why his wife shows no interest. When he tries asking her, she will not talk about it or give any explanation. The husband will grow frustrated, angry, and humiliated. He will feel that he has lost the comfort, shelter, and love in his home and that will lead to the chain of reactions that I have seen time and again: anger, separation, divorce.

But there is a simple solution for this libido issue. I have a patient, a dynamic fifty-two-year-old businesswoman, who is successful and financially independent. She has had many male partners, has enjoyed sex, and has had a great deal of fun and joy through those relationships. However, she never found the specific man she would like to marry. But something happened a year ago when she met a man she really loved. He was fifty-six, divorced, with two grown kids. They live together, but he will not commit to marriage. He will not tell her why, and she couldn't figure it out.

As I do with all my patients, I asked her about her sexual activity. She said that they have sex only once or twice a month. When I asked the reason, she said that in the past two years she has lost her libido. When I asked about her partner, she immediately said, "He has a strong sex desire and would love much more sex." This intelligent, successful, and sexually-experienced woman did not understand this important reality that was having a powerful impact on her life and happiness. She had become sexually paralyzed because of the loss of her libido.

I spoke with her like I have done with many other women. I told her that sex is a gift, and that she should never let it go. Engaging in sex will give her motivation, excitement, and youthful energy. Keeping her sexuality active will increase her passion and strengthen her femininity, her confidence, and her connection with her partner. She admitted to me that she had never thought that way about her libido. "It never occurred to me that my libido should not stop me from engaging in sex." I have heard this comment from many, many women when I discussed this issue with them! My patient responded to my talk immediately, became excited, and regained some of her confidence. I instructed her to exercise for five hours a week, count calories, and engage in sexual activity one or two times per week.

Four months later, this lady came back for a follow-up related to her exercise and weight loss. She appeared happy, excited, and trim. She hugged me and proudly waved her finger to show me her engagement ring! How can it be possible that this libido problem is allowed to cause us so much agony and harm while its solution is so simple and easy?

Finally, there's the perception that there is something wrong with men for wanting sex. Men's need for sex is normal and healthy, and while it may change with age, it usually remains strong. Because women often experience a loss of desire, lack of understanding causes them to look at men as sex maniacs who don't respect their wives. Nothing could be further from the truth. Men who hunger for sex are simply being men, and women should not judge them for that or make them beg for sex.

These are serious issues, but they can be overcome if women and men can take the time to learn how the other sex functions and understand the profound differences between the genders. The difference in how men and women function and get pleasure from sex is *not personal.* It is the way the genders are made. If men and women can consciously change how they view themselves and each other and be more open, cooperative, patient, and understanding, perhaps we can move past the crisis stage and on to lasting happiness.

Chapter Four

MEN AND ERECTILE DYSFUNCTION: A **CRISIS** OF SECRECY

I n the early days of medicine, the physicians of the time had some ideas about health and the causes of disease that were interesting, to say the least. One example was the condition known as *hysteria*, which was a catch-all for all kinds of alleged health problems experienced by women. A woman experiencing anything from depression to seizures might be diagnosed as being hysterical and "treated" with pseudo-therapies ranging from purging, toxic herbs, and in some cases, sexual orgies.[1] Calling this medicine was being generous.

Another condition subjected to this same quasi-mystical sort of guesswork was what was known in the seventeenth, eighteenth, and nineteenth centuries as impotence—what we call ED today. Despite grotesque therapies for ED that included electroshock and flogging, there are two things that are most telling to me about the outdated medical view of impotence. First, the word itself comes from the Latin word *impotencia*, which translates as "lack of power." That reflects the longstanding belief that a man who cannot engage in sexual intercourse at will is not virile—is not masculine.[2]

Second, while treatments for ED have changed completely with the advent of modern medicine, attitudes about it—especially among men—have changed very little. Call it impotence or ED, it still lies at the center of men's feelings of identity and masculinity. The failure to achieve or maintain an erection, perform sexually, or satisfy a partner can quickly become a psychological and emotional disaster for a man, leading to everything from problems with mental and physical health to damage to his marriage.

It is important that women and men understand what ED is, why it happens, what causes it, and how it can be treated, so that this very common condition does not cause harm to otherwise healthy marriages. That is the purpose of this chapter. Please keep in mind that the detrimental effects of ED are not just a problem for men but are equally a problem for the spouse. ED needs to be handled and resolved by both partners.

OPEN DISCUSSION ABOUT INTIMACY AND ITS POSITIVE EFFECT ON MARRIAGE

Let us look at this couple: the man was forty-five years old and the woman forty-one. They had been married for eleven years and had two beautiful kids. They had enjoyed a great marriage and good sex life until two years earlier, when the woman started to decline the man's sexual advances without much discussion. As you might expect for a healthy young man, her husband had a strong sexual drive and was humiliated that he had to ask for sex and be confronted with refusal.

Finally, he quit asking, and his resentment toward her grew. He became impolite, impatient, and short tempered. She responded with silence and a sour attitude, then became passive and barely spoke to him. The children saw this ugliness and developed nightmares, fear, and crying fits to the point that life started to become unbearable for the entire family. Then one day, she said she wanted to move out of the house and would ask for a divorce.

At that stage, the usual things we see started to happen. Both hired their own attorneys and began making plans to tear their family apart. Their luck changed when the wife showed up in my office asking for sleeping pills and antidepressants. I had known this couple as charming and happy, but when I asked her about her personal life, she told me sadly that she had started the process of divorce. She could not understand the reason; her husband had changed so much in the last year, and she said she feared that maybe something was not right with him. After I asked about their sexual relations, she admitted that they had not had sex for the past two years. When I asked why, she said that she cared less for sex because the care of their children was demanding and she just did not have the energy. She also said that she and her husband had never discussed this problem. Are you seeing the pattern here?

At that point, I spent a few minutes talking with her about basic sexuality, which she did not know much about. I explained the sexual needs of both men and women and told her that while she was so busy caring for the children, she had neglected herself and her marriage. I asked her if she would talk to her husband about their sex life before she saw her lawyer. I asked her to exercise five hours a week, and if that didn't help, to take the pills I gave her.

Three months later, when her husband came for his routine visit, he said, "Doc, what kind of pills did you give my wife? They worked a miracle on her." I asked him what he meant, and he said, "She's back to being the woman I met years ago." I learned from this couple, who I admired and respected, and I hope they will share their story with their kids when they are old enough. It is brave to speak about what is hidden inside your heart, and so often, it is the only medicine that you need.

SEXUAL ENERGY IS MASCULINE ENERGY

FOR THE MAN, SEXUAL POTENCY symbolizes nearly everything that he believes makes him a man. It represents his worldly ambition and passion to pursue his desires. It is a strong motivating factor in keeping fit, staying healthy, maintaining good grooming, and looking handsome as he ages. It represents his creativity—quite literally, since the ability to have sex is what allows a man to be part of the act of creating a child. And of course, it represents his ability to successfully pursue women and enjoy sexual conquest. Sexuality in a man is one of the main sources of his pride and motivation and has an important connection to his professional ambition and aspirations.

In other words, sexual potency is at the very core of the male identity, even for men who do not consider themselves to be "macho." Properly channeled, that belief can be a force for good. Virile, passionate, fiery men are forces for change and for doing great things, from landing on the moon to building great companies and inventing wonders like the internet.

However, the opposite is also true. Men who suffer from ED, even when it is caused by something like prostate cancer surgery that is out of their control, often suffer psychologically and emotionally. Research has shown that men with ED consistently reported feeling less masculine, like they were no longer men at all. They experienced higher levels of depression, embarrassment, and fear of being stigmatized by their peers and others.[3] Even for men who seem otherwise stable, mentally healthy, and well-adjusted, the perceived loss of their sexual self can be devastating.

This is the scenario I have seen over and over again: A man spends the evening with the woman he has been with for many years, and they try to have sex only to find that, for the first time, he cannot get an erection. As I have said, this is common, affecting about half of men over age forty. When it happens, his wife consoles him and goes to sleep; it may not be a big deal to her. But the man is alone in the dark, wondering about his capability, and there is no one to give him help or advice in dealing with the monstrous fear that this function—which is essential to his identity—is betraying him. If you are a young woman, imagine that you had just been told that you were infertile and could never bear children. How catastrophic would that feel to you? That is how men feel when ED ambushes them.

Let's look at this couple: He was forty-seven, and his wife was thirty-eight. They had been married for twelve years; both were professionals who made good money. He started to see me for blood pressure and neck problems, but he was a generally healthy man. Now he was unhappy, depressed, and not motivated to exercise. When I asked him about their sex life, he said that it was very good until two years ago. Now they had sex only about once a month. When I asked him for the reason, he said that his wife is very sexual and enjoys frequent sex. The reason sex was rare was because of him.

Two years before, he experienced a bad incident of ED, and since then he had developed persistent ED with his wife. He said, "I am ashamed and embarrassed because every time it happens, my wife becomes angry and agitated." Therefore, he avoided sex. Then, when he was on a business trip, he met a charming girl who was attracted to him, and they had sex. To his surprise, he performed as well as he had before his ED. That experience lit a fire in him, and he continued to have sex with various women, performing with pleasure and satisfaction. However, when he tried to have sex with his wife, it always ended with ED, humiliation, failure, anger, and blame.

When I asked what his plan was for the future, he said he was making preparations for divorce because he could not take it anymore. Up to that moment, he and his wife had never discussed sex with each other. She had no clue what he was planning. I have seen many couples like this one, and they have taught me that for men, ED is a true crisis. The majority of men experiencing it will try to hide it and search for excuses to handle the humiliation and guilt. But they will not talk to their wives.

ED IS PSYCHOLOGICAL

THE TERRIBLE ASPECT OF ALL this is that ED is, at its core, psychological. There are physiological causes, but about 70 percent of cases are due to anxiety—to fear. As you know, if you have a fear of something like heights or public speaking, that is a phobia. If you don't try to manage and control it, it will encroach negatively on your life and affect your behavior. Imagine the man facing the morning after his first instance of ED, and imagine how much anxiety he will feel about his next sexual encounter! He will feel shame, embarrassment, and truthfully, terror. This can damage his self-confidence, his behavior, his attitude toward his wife, and his future.

Approaching the next sexual encounter after the first failure, he will be loaded with fear and apprehension that it may happen again. Worse, he fears that it will become a pattern, and that enormous fear will invite the second failure, the third, and so on until the fear becomes a permanent mountain in front of him. He's lost. Who can he call for advice or guidance, and who can he talk to about something so shameful who will keep it a secret? I have seen these cases in large numbers, and I have seen the deterioration in men's physical and mental health because of something that to women can seem trivial.

However, ED is not trivial, and it's not just a problem for the man to deal with. I have seen ED destroy marriages and families, so this is very much a problem for the spouse to deal with as well.

My experience tells me that to a great degree, ED is a side effect of modern life. True, research is finding that even young men who suffer from ED are at higher risk of developing cardiovascular disease (CVD) later in life.[4] However, my clinical experience with thousands of men in middle age and older who have little or no CVD suggests that psychological factors loom large. I would agree, of course, that ED, CVD, diabetes, or neurological conditions can cause this disorder for some men. But when you consider the number of healthy, young men who experience this devastating problem, it's clear that it starts in the mind.

Sexual potency is linked to success in men's minds, and today's society places a great deal of pressure on men to succeed and dominate in all areas. Under this constant pressure, any man who fails at his career or being a financial success will feel inadequate compared to his peers and perceive himself as lacking power or strength. That creates the feeling of doubt that may translate into fear and nonperformance in the bedroom. I have observed men who retired from their work, particularly at a young age, but who had prepared no alternative goals and projects to give direction to their lives. Many of these men end up struggling with ED.

ED damages the male self-image as creator, predator, con-

FEAR AS A CAUSE OF ED IN MEN

My patient was a successful fifty-six-year-old man with a beautiful wife, who was his partner and a wonderful mother. Things were going well until we discovered that he had prostate cancer. He became very anxious and frightened about losing his sexual potency if he had surgery. On the other hand, surgery was his only treatment option. It took him six months to find the best prostate surgeon in the country, but following the surgery, he became anxious and obsessed with retaining his potency. However, despite all his effort and to his great disappointment, he developed ED and was not able to function sexually.

In the following eight months, he went to various urologists who started him on treatment with Viagra, vacuum devices, injections into the penis before sex, and more. But the more he tried, the worse the results were. Finally, a doctor gave him the option to have implant surgery. As you can imagine, this process was difficult for him and his wife. However, his wife turned out to be very practical and supportive. She was a real friend and ally to him during the whole ordeal and impressed me with her guidance and support. One day, after another treatment had failed and he was in despair, she advised him to stop all the treatments and turn back to nature. He decided to follow her advice, and without using any of the urologists' recommended treatments, within four weeks his sexual function began to return to normal. Before long, it was back to what it was before the surgery.

Was this a miracle? No. The key was that the man's stress, fear, and obsession over his lack of potency were *causing* his lack of potency. When he relaxed, he regained his ability to perform. This case shows that recommending complex treatments without taking into consideration the emotional component of ED is poor medical practice. Additionally, we are seeing the critical benefit of emotional support. I gave the wife guidance, but she took the lead. Her care and support made all the difference.

queror, and satisfier of all the needs of the flesh, from food to sex. It is, for most men, a psychological disorder with a physical symptom, in part because too many men define themselves by myths of sexual potency that have no ground in reality.

ED causes emotional trauma, shame, a sense of deficiency, and personal humiliation. The problem only grows when the spouse is ignorant about the facts behind ED and allows herself to believe that it is not her problem. She may wash her hands of it because she believes it is a man's issue. It would be a thousand times more helpful if she talked with her husband about his fears and then suggested he see his doctor. That is good advice, as this next case shows:

My patient was a forty-six-year-old African American man who came to me to treat his blood pressure and fatigue. He never mentioned anything about sex but stressed that he was not happy with his wife and that their relations had been strained. After I questioned him further, he told me about his ED. He had kept it a secret because he was ashamed and didn't want his wife to know about it. Therefore, he avoided sexual relations. He said, "A black woman will not respect her husband if he fails sexually." They were close to divorce. This man was really suffering and had no way solve his problems. Shame kept him from telling anybody, therefore, he could not get any help.

I found out that his previous doctor treated him for high blood pressure with beta-blockers, a medication that can cause or aggravate sexual disorders in men. I changed him to a different medication, and voilà! Shortly thereafter, he was able to function better, and by the time he regained his confidence, his sexual ability returned to normal. His relationship with his wife improved, and the family stayed together.

Canary in a Coal Mine for Heart Disease

*ED can be more than a cause for embarrassment; it can be an early
warning sign of cardiovascular disease, even in men who appear
otherwise healthy and have no obvious CVD risk factors. The reason is
simple: the penis is basically a hydraulic system. Blood flows into it to
make it erect, and when that blood flow is restricted by atherosclerosis,
or hardening of the arteries, that is a sign that blood flow elsewhere,
such as the coronary arteries, could be restricted as well. Men of any
age who are experiencing ED for the first time should see their physician for a full physical and bloodwork to identify potential CVD risk
factors. Early intervention can make a big difference.[5]*

*Still, the majority of my patients with ED have no evidence of CVD.
A physician needs to search for other reasons that may impair the
nervous system, like diabetes or thyroid or a testosterone deficiency.*

WHAT CAUSES ED?

IN MY OPINION, ED is an invention of the pharmaceutical
industry intended to help them sell billions of dollars' worth of
drugs like Viagra and Cialis. But since some cases of ED do have
legitimate physiological causes, the condition is not entirely in
men's heads. So how can it be a creation of Big Pharma?

Simply said, ED is a condition, but it is not a disease. It is
common to the point that about half of men will experience it
once they pass forty years of age. But calling it a disease is like
calling the sore knees of old age, a fever, or a headache a disease.
The "disease" is actually the terror, humiliation, isolation, and
loss of confidence that so many men feel after experiencing such a
common occurrence. With Big Pharma and advertisers egging us

on, we have turned ED into a psychological and emotional plague when it should be nothing more than something couples shrug over . . . and then talk to their physician about.

ED represents a functional disorder in the regulation of the autonomic nervous system, just like irritable bowel syndrome (IBS), overactive bladder, or hot flashes. The difference is that people approach disorders like IBS with understanding and confidence to learn how to handle them, while ED instead intrudes into the confidence, pride, and capability of a man to the point that it causes a chain reaction of other functional disorders that may throw the man into incapacity.

Therefore, it is essential for the physician to respect his patient's symptoms of ED and to try to understand its background and real cause and not just write a Viagra prescription. He should discuss the causes of ED clearly with the patient in such a manner that will remove the fear and the humiliation. Treating ED is like treating a fever. The physician might work to find the cause of the fever but will also treat it as a symptom and suggest aspirin. The smart physician will try to find the cause of ED but also treat the symptom with Viagra. It he comes to the conclusion that the ED is psychological, he will treat it as such while using Viagra to rebuild the patient's confidence.

The disease is the perception that "real men don't get ED"—that so-called "real men" can get a rock-hard erection on command, and a man who can't, even once, for any reason, is less than a man. That thinking is behind the terrible secret anxiety that most men experience after just one failure, and it leads to further failure, turning ED into a self-sustaining cycle of shame.

What causes ED? There are many possible causes:

- *Physical* causes such as early stage CVD, hypertension, an enlarged prostate, prostate cancer treatment, high cholesterol, type 2 diabetes, insomnia, smoking, the use of alcohol or other drugs, an injury to the penis, low testosterone levels or other hormonal problems like low thyroid, spinal cord injury, and some medications, such as those taken for blood pressure and clinical depression (which also can affect libido). However, these purely physiological factors account for only about 30 percent of the ED cases that PCPs see in our offices.

- The majority of ED cases are *psychological*. There is no underlying physical pathology that could account for the man's inability to perform. Anything from relationship problems, job stress, and fatigue, to not finding your partner physically attractive, anxiety, and depression can cause the man to fail to get an erection. Even heavy use of online pornography, research has shown, can impair a man's ability to achieve an erection because an interaction with a real woman does not activate his brain's "reward circuitry" in the same way that porn does.[6]

The thing is, as complex and sensitive as the mechanism that leads to erections is, we should expect failures from time to time even in a healthy man. In reality, it is the men who *never* fail to achieve erections who are the exceptions, not the men who experience ED once in a while when tired or stressed out! When a man is in emotional distress, fatigued, or distracted, or when there are hormonal changes that normally occur with age, ED will happen from time to time. I have heard this from men who are as young as twenty-five years old: "Well, when I'm tired, or when she is angry with me, I just can't get it up. It doesn't want to work."

We also need to keep in mind that the process of erection is not voluntary. It is regulated by a complex physiological process attached to numerous physical systems, and little disturbances in one or more systems will disturb its efficacy. However, above all, the mental status of the man is important.

Contributing to this problem is the importance our culture has attached to the idea of a man being a sex machine because men believe they must conform to this stereotype. Let's say a typical man fails to achieve an erection with his wife one time out of thirty encounters. Pretty good, right? Not for the man. That one failure will loom a thousand times larger in his mind than the twenty-nine successes, even if those other occasions all ended with his wife feeling deeply satisfied. It will haunt him and may throw him into a negative chain reaction that will start a complex process.

What do you think that man will feel like when he goes to work the next day? He will think, *Something is wrong with me.* He will be tentative, unsure, doubtful of his abilities. That fear, shame, and sense of emasculation is the true cause of ED—and it can be overcome, usually with ease.

Much will depend on how the man's spouse responds at that critical moment. For that reason, we should educate women and explain the facts about ED. If women are aware of the enormous emotional toll that even a single incident of ED can have on their partner, they can be better prepared to respond constructively and supportively to what is most likely to be perceived as a crisis in the partner's mind.

TAKING AWAY THE FEAR

THIS IS WHY THE FIRST thing I do when I meet with male patients who are experiencing ED is tell them how common ED really is. I say, "Take your age and convert it to a percentage, and that is the percentage of the time you may expect to fail to get an erection on the first try." Their eyes get wide; no one has ever told them this. If you are forty years old, four times out of ten you may fail to get an erection without extra stimulation, and this is normal. That knowledge changes everything for these anxious men. They had been assuming there was something terribly wrong with them, and I've told them there is not. "But," I also say, "if you turn your worry into a phobia that you are impotent and have some terrible disease, then you will fail 100 percent of the time."

What happens when the desire is there, but the penis does not get erect? It may happen due to stress, fatigue, alcohol, drugs, a physical cause, or a conflict in the relationship, but we should not label it as a disease. Suppose you slept on your arm and compressed the nerve feeding that arm long enough to put it to sleep. You wake up and find out that your arm is numb. You might panic, thinking that you have had a stroke. Similarly, when a man realizes that his erection is not happening, his first reaction is usually to panic and assume something is terribly wrong.

This is not true. ED does not mean desire is not present. It doesn't mean the man doesn't want sex. Men want sex even in the complete and permanent absence of the ability to achieve an erection. Some men will even reach orgasm with very little erection.

I also let my male patients know that there are many ways to define ED and that an immediate failure doesn't mean sex is impossible. Technically, ED is the inability to get or sustain an erection long enough to have sexual intercourse. The trouble is that so many men become so humiliated after their initial failure to perform that they stop trying in order to avoid failure and shame. They are unaware that there are options and that the fear is the real problem. The more they surrender to it, the worse the result will be.

There are several commonsense solutions. First of all, if couples regarded ED less as a catastrophe and more as an, "Oops, well, that didn't work out!" situation, they would take a break and try something else to help the man achieve an erection—other kinds of stimulation, erotic talk, cuddling, and any number of other means to get the man aroused. But when men and women react to an episode of ED as though the world has just ended, the problem only gets worse. The key really lies with how the woman responds on the scene. We should educate all women about male sexual function and how they can respond to an episode of ED helpfully and constructively.

Second, just because the man experiences this common problem does not mean he cannot satisfy the woman. Remember, most women do not climax through intercourse. Oral sex, manual stimulation, and vibrators are all options that the man can use that will leave his partner feeling good and very satisfied.

It is also critical for men with ED to see their doctors and learn that they are not impaired. Yes, there are many possible physiological causes of ED, but almost all are treatable. I will reassure the patient (as well as myself) by checking all other physical factors that can affect sexual function, like the circulatory and nervous systems, but in the majority of cases the most important part of their body to fix is their head. This is how I know: the majority of men with ED avoid sexual encounters with women, but they tell me that they always achieve normal erection, orgasm, and satisfaction through masturbation. That's a clear indication to me that they are physically fine! If you get a normal erection during masturbation, you are completely normal, and need only to clear your head of the fear.

This is especially true of young men who can't believe this is happening to them. They feel betrayed and old before their time. They are scared. I remind them that pills can help, and exercise and improving their general health will be beneficial. Anything that improves circulation, boosts testosterone levels, and enhances their body image will help both the body and mind.

By the time I get through telling men this, their fear is usually diminished. They've heard from a professional that their life is not over—that there is hope. There are ways to treat and manage this, and they are not alone. That's the big thing. They've come to me dreading intimate time with their partner. Sometimes, they reject their partners because they fear being embarrassed, and this just leads the woman to feel hurt and suspicious. They come to my office loaded with guilt, shame, embarrassment, and a shattered ego, all of which will usually not surface until I ask about their sex life. After a candid ten- to fifteen-minute talk about all these things, they are like new men, and I haven't given them a pill, they haven't run a second on a treadmill, and they haven't lost an ounce.

This is why treating ED starts with treating the fears about it as well as making men aware of all the heavy cultural baggage they have been carrying around. Even when ED has a legitimate physical cause such as diabetes or hypertension, too many men won't seek treatment for those conditions because they are embarrassed. That's bad for their overall health as well as their sex life. When we get rid of the stigma, we make treatment an option.

ED CAN ALWAYS BE TREATED

MEDICATIONS CAN BE CHANGED, chronic conditions can be treated, and if ED persists, there are sexual workarounds. The key thing to remember here, as with the overall question of whether a husband and wife have to resign themselves to a life without sex, is this:

> *There is hope for men with ED. If a man is willing to talk to his physician and his wife and get past the emotional trauma associated with ED, there are options. The odds are good that he can function again sexually, satisfy his wife, and keep a happy marriage.*

Take this example of another patient of mine: This man was forty-eight years old and married. His wife was forty-four, and they were healthy. But their marriage was not happy. He was very concerned about his wife having an affair. He came to me for his blood pressure, but when I asked, "How is your marriage?" he opened up to me. He admitted that during the past year, he had experienced problems maintaining an erection. He never told anybody, but frequently he had to quit in the middle of sex, which embarrassed him very much. He had no idea what to do. He was terrified that something was wrong with him and was consumed with fear and worry.

He was also worried about his wife sleeping with another man because she was still interested in being active sexually. The trouble was the secrecy. He had never discussed this problem with anybody—not me, not his wife, not close friends—because he felt such embarrassment and failure. The taboo blocked him from seeking help, discussing his problem with a professional, or being comforted by friends. He was left alone, isolated and miserable. In my experience, secrecy, isolation, and the sense of being alone with a health problem cause as much damage and pain as the health problem itself. That is certainly true of ED. But once I asked him about his sex life, I broke that barrier. It had started one year earlier and only gotten worse, and as a result he avoided sex with his wife, using all kinds of excuses in order to guard his pride.

I told him that the first thing we would do was examine the three systems behind sexual potency—neurological, circulatory, and endocrine—to prove to him that he was normal. I did this, and I found nothing wrong with him. No liver disease, kidney disease, or heart disease. He wasn't taking any medication that could cause ED. Then I told him, "There is nothing wrong with you. You can do this."

I prescribed Viagra, and he took it. He trusted me because I dealt with a very sensitive issue for him in a candid, logical, and respectful way, and he listened and felt like I was his ally. It was obvious that this man was preoccupied with his sexual failure and that had induced more failure. It's the quote, "The only thing we have to fear is fear itself" in real life. I said to him, "Start with Viagra, and in six months the whole thing will change." In six months, he came back and told me, "I rarely use the Viagra now. To tell you the truth, doctor, I think I do well without it."

So did he invent this disease, or was it real? The answer to both questions is yes. Whether ED is physical or psychological, it only becomes a disease when men (and women) treat it as a cause for fear, panic, paranoia, and shame. When that happens, anxiety makes the man develop ED as a sort of hysterical paralysis. If men can break the secrecy and speak out openly, none of that pain is necessary.

Incidentally, there are two types of ED in the medical literature: the one where the man fails to reach erection, and the other where the man develops an erection that quickly ends with premature ejaculation. Both are traumatic. The second type of ED can be a problem because the male erection is brief and the woman's orgasm is delayed, so the man feels unable to sexually satisfy his wife, which seems like a cruel joke. Such physiological events are normal with age, and even premature ejaculation is treatable if the man trains his neurological response. But since they are usually not discussed or dealt with, they create emotional defeat for both partners and often lead to emotional and medical problems.

With my patients, I have learned how to get men talking about both types of ED and to advise them on changing how they handle this self-destructive, mostly psychological disorder. Just opening the conversation with understanding provides great relief. I instruct them how to train themselves to delay their orgasm and prolong their erection. A person can train the involuntary physiological systems through the mind and certain exercises, just as with yoga and meditation one can lower the pulse and blood pressure. It's not that different from training babies to control their bowel and bladder functions as they get older, even though these functions are not controlled by our voluntary systems.

I also explain how, when they can't maintain an erection, men can continue to stimulate their wives and bring them to orgasm, helping them continue to feel masculine. The ability to satisfy their partners takes away a lot of men's fears.

WHAT MEN CAN DO

THERE ARE SOME MEN WHO handle the loss of potency well. I have a patient who is eighty years old. Twenty-five years ago, he underwent open abdominal prostatectomy to remove his prostate because of cancer. Back then, they didn't know how to spare the nerve that helps the penis achieve arousal, so he became organically impotent.

Initially, he accepted that verdict. But we started to talk about how he could still satisfy his wife sexually using manual stimulation. And to his credit, he listened and did it. Finally, she turned eighty herself and told him that she didn't really care about sex anymore. But despite all his health problems, they still have a happy marriage. They are always together, hugging and holding hands. Life is good for them, and I'm sure that part of it is due to the fact that they figured out how to enjoy sexuality without the erection. Open communication unlocks the door to enjoying life together even when there are problems with sexual function.

When they finally open up to their partner and physician about ED, men can take many steps that can restore their sexual performance and the harmony and closeness in their relationship. Everything starts, of course, with a comprehensive physical examination and consultation with a doctor. That medical evaluation, followed by open and candid discussion between doctor and patient, determines what needs to be done to resolve the problem. With that information in hand, these are some of the things men can do:

- **Exercise regularly.** I recommend regular exercise for all my patients because regular exercise is the closest thing we have to a fountain of youth. For men, who are more susceptible at a younger age than women to heart disease, regular workouts improve circulation, control weight, boost testosterone levels, increase energy, help control blood sugar—you name it. Ideally, try to do a blend of aerobic exercise and strength training, but even regular walking is beneficial. A 2007 study published in *Harvard Men's Health Watch* found that just thirty minutes of daily walking reduced men's risk of ED by 41 percent.[7] When circulation increases during exercise, it does so in all parts of the body, including the sexual organs, adding more nutrition and stimulation to that system.

- **Eat a healthy diet.** The Massachusetts Male Aging Study, a massive study of men conducted over two years in and around Boston, found that men who ate high amounts of vegetables, fruit, whole grains, and fish while avoiding red meat and heavily processed foods experienced less ED.[8]

- **Pay attention to heart health.** I have already mentioned that the erection depends on healthy blood flow and the release of vasodilators (compounds that expand the blood vessels) like nitric oxide. So it makes sense that if a man who wants to avoid or cure ED, should take good care of his cardiovascular system. That means, among other things, maintaining healthy blood pressure, cholesterol and triglyceride levels, getting regular checkups, and ensuring that if there are signs of CVD, they are addressed through lifestyle changes, medication, or both.

- **Keep weight under control.** About 25 percent of new cases of ED today are in men under age forty, which was rare in the past. This might have something to do with the population's overall testosterone levels dropping in the last thirty years due to an increase in obesity.[9] A man with a larger waistline is more likely to have ED than a slimmer man, for many reasons. Obesity increases blood sugar levels, raising diabetes risk. It causes inflammation throughout the body, which constricts blood vessels. Fat disrupts hormone levels. But if you exercise and follow a healthy diet, the weight should come off, and many other negative metabolic effects of being overweight will improve as well.

- **Stop smoking.** Men who smoke are more likely to experience ED because smoking causes blood vessels to constrict while contributing to blockage by plaque.[10] Anyway, smoking is one of the worst things you can do for your health, period. Quit.

- **Manage stress.** Chronic stress is as bad as smoking for your heart, circulatory system, and brain. The constant flood of cortisol and adrenaline reduces blood flow, affects the levels of neurotransmitters in the brain, and wrecks sleep. Find ways to reduce or eliminate stress, whether that means meditation, yoga, exercise, relaxation, or radical steps like changing jobs. Most of all, get seven to eight hours of good sleep. This is important to all your health systems. Do not trade good, sound sleep for the best treasure on earth.

- **Take supplements.** There are a few dietary supplements that have been tested for their efficacy in helping ED, and some have shown promise. DHEA, the amino acid l-arginine, and Panax ginseng may be of help.[11] However, I would advise you to be cautious in general when considering taking supplements. Some may interact with medicine you're currently taking, while others are a waste of money.

But more important than all this is to talk about it. Socially, ED is shrouded in secrecy. Men don't talk about it, even to other men, and research shows that 70 percent of men don't talk about ED with their physicians, even when they have symptoms. This must change if men are to get relief from the fear and shame that can ruin their lives.

Take this case of mine: a man, fifty-two years old, married for twenty-seven years. His wife was fifty, and they had three grown children. For the past four years, they had had no sexual relations. They slept in different rooms because he snores. He had gained forty-two pounds and did not exercise because of poor energy and fatigue. When I asked about his sexual life, he was willing to tell me that he was not happy with himself because he masturbated, but he would not approach his wife for sex because he had ED and was afraid of being humiliated.

This man was depressed and kept gaining weight. Following my medical investigation, I found him to have sleep apnea and prescribed a CPAP (continuous positive airway pressure) machine, which helps breathing during sleep. Finally getting better sleep, the man had more energy, and he began to exercise and lost weight. As a result, he didn't need the CPAP anymore, regained his sexual potency, and began having sex with his wife again. They became close to each other, traveling, enjoying sex twice a week, and living as a happy couple.

Imagine if this man had continued to keep his ED a secret. It would have continued to have a negative effect on his life, marriage, and health.

ED Treatment for the Man and the Woman

It is natural to think of ED as strictly a male problem. However, that does not make sense in the context of a relationship. Research shows that when women are with a man experiencing ED, the impact on the relationship varies widely. Some women feel hopeless and helpless about their future sex lives; others are able to support their husbands and find new ways to be intimate that persist even after the man regains his potency. The consensus is clear: when a man experiences ED, treatment should include the woman, too.[12] She should know why this is happening, that it is not a reflection on her sexuality, how she can and should support her husband, and what can be done to correct the problem. This will improve the odds that the couple stays together and enjoys happy relations.

ED is a problem that both husband and wife should handle together, instead of just the wife blaming herself that she is not attractive enough to be desirable or blaming her man for being unable to satisfy her.

HOW ED AFFECTS WOMEN

IN EIGHTEENTH-CENTURY ENGLAND, THERE WERE at least thirty-two documented cases where women sued their husbands for failing to consummate their marriages due to impotence.[13] The trials were scandalous affairs, but they revealed the importance of male potency and power not only to the man but to women as well.

As we work to help couples deal with the changes to sexuality that come with age, it is vital that women understand their role in dealing with ED and not let it destroy their self-confidence and relationships. Throughout history and today, ED affects women. My practice has shown me that the effect of ED on the woman can be nearly as devastating as it is on the man.

Imagine that you are a woman married to the same man for twenty-five years. You love this man, find him sexy and attractive, and have rarely had a sexual complaint. Then one night, he cannot perform. You make light of the problem, saying, "It's okay, honey; we'll try again in the morning," and go to sleep. But the problem escalates. Your man lies awake all night wondering what is wrong and feeling humiliated at not being able to satisfy you. In the morning, he still can't perform. If this continues, you grow concerned and sexually frustrated and watch him distance himself from you, becoming cold or short tempered. After a while, you don't even recognize this man, and you have no idea what to do or how to help. You might even start thinking about divorce!

This is not simply a matter of the relationship, either. Research has shown that when a woman's partner experiences ED, her own libido, arousal, frequency of orgasm, and overall satisfaction with sex goes down as well.[14] This is in part because, unlike men whose sex drive remains strong for most of their lives even with ED, women's libido is more of a "use it or lose it" proposition. (I'll explore this more in the next chapter.) The more sexually active she is, the more she feels desired, and the happier she is sexually and emotionally, the more the average woman *wants* and *enjoys* sex. If her husband is terrified of failure, humiliated by ED, or shunning his wife because he's angry and frustrated, her desire will mirror his. Both will be unhappy and resentful.

So it is essential for women to recognize that they have a great deal of power and responsibility in this situation, for better or worse. First, women must understand how vulnerable men can be regarding their potency. A woman might not think her husband *should* place such importance on whether or not he can get an erection, but men *do* attach such importance to this. ED can be devastating to a man's self-esteem, and the woman must respect that for many men ED is an identity crisis. Therefore, it is essential that women understand and learn the factors behind their man's sexuality and become familiar with how she can help things improve.

HOW WOMEN CAN HELP

THE WOMAN'S ROLE IN DEALING with ED in a productive way begins with two choices. First, when the man experiences ED for the first time, the woman should not make light of it or joke about it. She cannot be critical or distance herself from the issue. This could damage the couple's sex life and cause irreparable damage to their marriage because the man feels deep shame. The woman should also not act as though a single episode of ED is an emergency, making the man feel that there is something wrong with him.

The right way to approach the issue is with calm and maturity: acknowledge it, talk about how sex can continue during that encounter, be supportive and encouraging, and express faith and belief in the man's masculinity and past sexual prowess.

If the episode doesn't repeat, that is all the woman needs to do. Occasional ED is normal and expected. But if the man fails repeatedly, the woman should not allow the issue to fester and remain secret. Men often feel great shame over ED, and if the man hides from everyone, that shame will grow, leading to broken self-confidence and emotional problems. Women are often willing to acknowledge ED before their partners will, and this allows them to talk openly and encourage the man to express his thoughts and worries.

The woman can also go with the man to see a physician to look into possible causes for the trouble. Research has shown that outcomes in managing ED are better when both partners are involved, and women have important parts to play, including:

- getting men to see their physician, which many men are reluctant to do

- assisting in getting necessary information to the physician and other professionals

- helping the man with therapies and lifestyle changes

- collaborating in changing the couple's sexual practices

- providing emotional support and encouragement[15]

Another important thing women can do when dealing with a man with ED is to make him aware that her sexual satisfaction is not the same as his. Remember, only about one-quarter of women reach orgasm through intercourse, but most men do not know this. There are many other ways a man can bring his wife to orgasm that don't require an erection, and knowing this can help the man feel less pressure, allow him to satisfy his wife, and keep his pride and self-esteem while he works his way through treatment and lifestyle changes.

Bottom line: ED is common and treatable, and it does not have to mean the end of a healthy marriage and wonderful sex life.

THERE IS ALWAYS HOPE

HOPE IS THE MESSAGE I will come back to again and again in this book. There is hope for couples with sexual problems and for couples facing the stress and shame of ED. However, that hope hinges on one thing:

> *Stop making ED a shameful secret.*
> *It may just be in your head.*

Hope begins when couples talk openly with each other about ED and its implications, and then talk with their physician, preferably as a couple. I seldom see women accompanying their husbands to the doctor, and that should become more common. Women who are part of the ED conversation are more knowledgeable and better prepared. Treatment works better, and it lightens the burden of the problem on the man.

When men suffer silently and in isolation, the problem only becomes worse. ED undermines men's confidence and self-worth. The relationship will suffer due to his guilt, shame, and anxiety. He will not pursue sex with his partner because he is terrified that she will judge him, and he will be embarrassed. Instead, he will avoid sexual contact with his wife and may masturbate to satisfy his sexual needs. He might drink or use drugs to deal with the anxiety, seek extramarital sex to avoid judgment, or try to reclaim his masculinity through impulsive, aggressive, or even violent behavior. I have seen it all.

Remember, men have a biological need for sex, and sexual pursuit, satisfaction, and potency play a critical role in male identity. That means that ED without the hope of successful treatment will undermine a man's self-worth and self-esteem. He will suffer and so will those around him. He will internalize the guilt and shame, which will impair his drive, ambition, work, energy level, and interest in life. He will conclude not only that something is wrong with him but that he is "less than a man" and a failure.

One of my female patients shared with me her enormous fear about her husband, who was not my patient. She told me she was frightened because her husband was becoming "crazy" as a result of his ED. It developed three years earlier, and he became paranoid and frustrated. First he blamed her for it, but then he blamed his previous doctor who treated him with blood pressure pills that he was sure had ruined his sex life. The woman told me that her husband became obsessed with that doctor and expressed anger and hatred toward him. Recently, he had purchased a gun and said that he might kill that doctor.

I told her that she should report him to the police. She replied, "God, if I report him to the police, he will shoot me instead because he was angry at me about his ED, too." I thought, *Does someone have to get shot to resolve ED?* Sexual frustration among men has no logic or common sense but can be wild, powerful, and destructive. I would advise all women to recognize that ED and sexual problems can cause irrational behavior in men, and to learn about it, become familiar with it, and help their partner to manage it effectively.

Secrecy and silence will ruin a man who is emotionally suffering from ED—along with the people close to him who may become affected by his mood and changes in behavior. The solution begins with open, compassionate, mature communication and with recognizing that ED is not a disease. It is not a defect. It is not a personal failure or a sign of a lack of masculinity. It is a common, normal condition that can almost always be treated, improved, and overcome. Talk about it with your doctor, and with your partner.

Chapter Five

WHY WOMEN SHOULD TREAT SEX LIKE GOING TO THE GYM

A while ago, I had the kind of sad experience in my office that this book is intended to prevent. I saw a male patient, forty-eight years old, very nice, and married to a forty-two-year-old woman. They have three children, but after the last child was born three years earlier, his wife lost all her interest in sex. Their relationship stayed outwardly the same, except that there was no sex. When the man tried to approach his wife about sex, she told him that she would not do anything that she had no interest in, and she declined to have any further discussion on the matter.

The man was angry, confused, and frustrated and was masturbating to get some relief from his urges. That day in my office, he admitted to me that he had finally decided to divorce his wife because he could not do anything to remedy the situation, and he was unwilling to continue a life without sex. It was terrible: his heart was broken, he knew his young kids would suffer, and he acknowledged that his wife was a good mother and a good woman. Could this family have been saved by what I've written here? I don't know. But I wish I had the opportunity to see this woman individually, as perhaps I could have persuaded her to look at the issue in a different way that could have led to a better outcome.

Between 25 to 63 percent of all women will experience some level of periodic sexual dysfunction,[1] and a smaller percentage will simply lose all interest in sex. But is it a final verdict written in stone that once libido is lost, it be lost forever? Medical science really doesn't understand why libido is lost in the first place (even among young women) with devastating consequences. What we do know is that low libido—not *frigidity,* a word that is just as outdated as *impotence*—is common among women, and when it is left untreated, it can cause critical damage to the woman's marriage and life.

There are not many reliable and confirmed treatments for low female libido, though some medications have shown promise, and psychotherapy appears to be helpful to some women.[2] One of the reasons I have written this book is that I believe that changing how women think about the role of sex in their marriages—and about what it means to agree to sex initially without libido—can change a great deal about how women see themselves. It can also change how they respond to their husbands' desire for sex.

Here's the key: I have seen women who engage in open discussions about sex and who agree to engage in sexual activity *despite* having low or no libido regain some or all of their sexual drive and revive the closeness and love of their relationships. Let us look at what that means.

I had a patient, fifty years old, a mother to two teenagers, and a wife to a successful husband. I found her to be in excellent health, but something looked missing in her life: the zest and sparkle that usually glitter in the eyes of happy person. When I asked her about her sex life, she said she and her husband hadn't had sex for a couple of years. I inquired further, and she appeared perplexed. This told me that she and her spouse had never talked to each other about sex. She said, "To tell you the truth, Doc, we don't know the answer. We both apparently lost our interest in sex, but we love each other, and we love our kids."

I asked her whether her husband had ever failed in his sexual performance and whether he tried to approach her sexually. She said she believed that he must have lost interest without having discussed it with him. This couple fell into a routine in which they ignored the reward and joy of emotional and physical intimacy. But this was not surprising to me. In making inquiries into people's private sexual lives, I have come to expect sexual problems built on secrecy, lack of communication, and blind acceptance, and I have found them to be undiagnosed and unrecognized in almost every couple. Mostly, couples are aware when things are not going well in their relationship although they often cannot identify the problem, let alone find a solution.

This charming lady needed direction and encouragement, so I asked her to take a vacation with her husband somewhere they could spend private time together, talk openly about sex, and engage in sexual activity. A few weeks later, the woman came back to review her blood tests. First, she thanked me for opening the discussion about their sexual lives. She started to tell how she enjoyed her short island vacation with her husband, how they walked on the beach, held hands, and watched the sunset. Best of all, they had sex every evening. Then she said, "I thought that my husband had lost his interest in sex, but he just gave up on me. Now life is so sweet for both of us, and how foolish we were not to see it."

I could see that this same lady was now feeling such peace and contentment. The sparkle in her eyes told me I had done a good job with this couple. Before she left my office, she scheduled her husband for an appointment as a new patient.

RESEARCH ISN'T THE SAME AS REAL LIFE

ACCORDING TO WORK BY THE Mayo Clinic, about 10 percent of women can be formally diagnosed with hypoactive sexual desire disorder (HSDD), which means that these women have no sexual desire or interest and no spontaneous arousal or sexual fantasies. Scientists think this problem could be caused by imbalances of hormones or neurotransmitters in the brain, but they are not sure. Treatment ideas are just as uncertain and include medication and cognitive behavioral therapy.[3] When you read between the lines of such research, you can almost see the frustrated shrugs. How about taking nature in its own dignity and glory and just follow where it leads?

In other words, the female libido is complicated, we don't understand why it stops working, and we don't have a lot of good information on how to treat it. We do know that many women treated with hormones like estrogen and testosterone say that they

HOW LACK OF COMMUNICATION CAN DAMAGE THE LIVES OF COUPLES

This was an incredible couple I treated: a man, thirty-eight, married to his teenage sweetheart for seventeen years. After I asked him during his visit, he confessed that their sexual relations were very rare—perhaps once every two months—but that when it happened, it was very good for both of them. The problem was that his wife had declined to respond to his advances for the last fifteen years. The problem started gradually, but now she would not discuss sex with him at all. Reluctantly, he turned to masturbation once or twice a week, but he had never gone to another woman because that was against his beliefs. That day, he asked me to talk to her.

I met with this nice young lady, who I know was devoted and loving. She said that the trouble had started fifteen years before when she noticed her libido diminishing. When she had a hysterectomy ten years earlier, the problem became worse. Now she only had the desire for sex four or five times a year. That was the only time she had sex. But when she did engage in sex, it was very good, and she achieved orgasm. When I asked why she was not responding to her husband, she gave me the same answer I heard from others, which is that she didn't have the drive at the moment when he approached her. She had never talked to anybody about this, neither professionals nor friends. However, it was her belief that a woman should not act sexually when her libido was not driving her.

After a lengthy discussion, I advised her to respond to her husband and get engaged in sexual activity as frequently as one to two times a week, even if she did not have the desire at the time sex was initiated. She appeared greatly relieved and excited about the idea. As she left, I thought, *What a waste of fifteen years—years of unhappiness for this couple.* However, I was encouraged that those fifteen years of silence and resentment were reversed with just talk, encouragement, and guidance.

CASE STUDY

feel significant improvement. However, some also claim to feel the same improvement from a placebo. The problem with these studies is that they rely on surveying women who understand their libido well enough to know when it is low and when is healthy. Plus, these surveys use standardized questions in printed form that treat the sexual system like it's a machine rather than dealing with the whole woman as a person with many interconnected systems, as well as a mind and a soul.

I have found that most women simply remain silent, accept their loss of desire, and expect their husbands to do the same. That is where research has its limitations. If you don't ask every woman you see in your office about her sexual function, you will not know how common this disorder is. This is exactly what I have done over forty-five years of practicing medicine and why I want to share it.

When a patient first comes to see him, the physician doesn't know if she has high blood pressure or diabetes unless she tells him. If she doesn't know either, the physician has to find answers himself by doing things like taking blood pressure measurement and getting blood work done. The same situation exists for sexual disorders, but worse. If the patient keeps it a secret and never tells the physician, he will never know of the sexual problem because there is no test that can detect it. Everyone will be in the dark.

However, when a physician proactively includes questions about sexuality in his routine medical questions, as I have been doing, then he will know. Through the years I came to realize that people are not only willing to free themselves from the secrecy and taboo, they are *eager* to. My patients have always answered my questions willingly, which tells me that they have been in great need of someone to listen to them about their sexual fears. They have also been eager to learn any suggestions or guidance that would improve their sexual life. This is why it is much more valuable to talk to people instead of having them fill out a questionnaire.

WOMEN SHOULD WELCOME THEIR SEXUALITY

THE LIBIDO IS LIKE THE appetite for food: it can change from day to day. The trouble begins when women assume that one bad day means desire is gone forever. If a woman does, she will build on the wrong assumption and begin to live her life without sexuality. That is the wrong way to go for any woman. It is against the feminine character, it is against her physical and emotional needs, it is against her own well-being, and it is against the well-being of her husband and family. If a woman surrenders to the negative forces pushing her to accept a life without sex, she may say to herself, "I am in a comfortable position, so my husband should just accept life without sex, and everyone will be happy."

That is a recipe for suffering. First, as we have discussed, men are not like women. Men *need* sex, and depriving them of it is a sure path to anger, conflict, and alienation. But while they are not the same as men, women also thrive when they enjoy sexual pleasure! It is a gift that adds excitement, charm, and glitter to life. A woman who becomes an asexual being is cutting herself off from all of that. The true tragedy is that none of that is necessary, but there is no one guiding women and telling them "Things do not have to be this way." So millions of women become victims of the cultural taboo of talking about sex, when in reality it should be discussed alongside any other health issues, such as diabetes, blood pressure heart conditions, kidney disfunction, and so on.

I wonder if women have accepted the idea that wanting sexual comfort and happiness in their marital life means they are less worthy of respect in their roles as mothers and wives. I would like to teach women that loving sex and finding joy in sexuality is not something they have to do for the sake of men. Women's sexuality belongs to them, not the men in their lives! But sexuality is not a "take it or leave it" proposition for women. Sex is part of a normal, vibrant, and physically and emotionally healthy life, and I encourage women to respect it—to attach as much importance to it as they do to equal pay and position with men. Women need and deserve equality, but they also should not neglect the need for warmth, desire, romance, and sexual satisfaction.

In fact, when it comes to sex in the bedroom, women have all the power. Men should take care of and respect women because they bring sensitivity, tenderness, and love to the world for all of us. We care for them by loving them, treating them with tenderness and respect, taking seriously their concerns about things like consent and sexual harassment, and helping them to feel seen, heard, and safe in every way.

Another way men can help women is to encourage them to enjoy their sexuality even in later life. This is why it's important for women to speak with their personal physician about their sexuality. In my practice, if I hear a woman saying, "I just have no interest in sex anymore," I explain her sexual physiology and her partner's and encourage her not to use libido as a gatekeeper to sex. I remind her that sex is a gift, not a burden or something she has to do for her husband. It is a privilege to enjoy sex and share it with her partner, so she should not let it go without a fight. I try to get my female patients to make sex a priority, even while their minds are preoccupied with daily duties like jobs or raising children.

Many women have told me that once they got past the barrier of lower libido by persuading themselves to keep going and hold on to their sexuality, their libido did return, and sexual satisfaction returned with it. They became aroused again, and many reached orgasm. So I would tell ladies that there is no reason why low libido has to stop a woman from enjoying a wonderful, sexually satisfying life.

Consider if you lost your desire to exercise or cook your meals. You would have two options: give in to the lack of desire and not cook a meal or exercise. The result will be unpleasant: you would gain weight and become unhealthy from getting no physical activity and eating packaged or junk foods. With the second option, you ignore the lack of desire and force yourself to go for exercise or cook healthy meals because you know both are good for you. Over time, you will feel better, look better, and be healthier by doing this even though *your lack of desire would have stopped you* if you had given into it.

When it comes to sex, women should also take the second option.

WHAT SEX MEANS TO WOMEN

ONE REASON IT IS SO hard to identify a cause for female low libido is that for women, sex is much more about the mind and emotion. For men, sex tends to be about conquest, but for women, it signifies femininity, closeness, being desirable, and the

THE EFFECT OF AN UNHEALTHY LIFESTYLE ON SEX AND HAPPINESS

The male patient was fifty-eight and married to his wife, fifty-two, for twenty years. No kids. They both were trim, beautiful, and happy. Their sexual relations were compatible, and they seemed like a happy couple. Then, eight years ago, things started to change. They both began gaining weight, chain smoking, and drinking and became unhappy and depressed.

I worked hard to help them change their bad habits. They tried hard to change, but they kept going in circles. They would change their bad habits, lose weight, and reduce smoking, but it was all temporary. Eventually, they would return to those bad habits. When I asked the woman about their sex life, she confirmed that it had almost ceased. She said, "Because he is not attracted to me anymore. I am fat and ugly." Her libido was still very good, but since he was not approaching her, she had resorted to masturbation and was very unhappy.

I confronted her husband separately and asked about their sex life. He said that he still had the interest but had experienced several episodes of ED and had decided not to approach his wife anymore because of the humiliation. He had started masturbating as well. They never discussed this with each other! They both felt unhappy, feeling worthless and guilty, and they had turned to destructive habits out of sexual frustration.

I was determined to help this couple, and that did not mean giving them anti-anxiety and antidepressant medication. Instead, I focused on their sexuality. First, I opened a conversation with the husband. I explained to him that the best avenue to stopping his unhealthy habits was to go back to sexual normalcy. I explained to him that ED is a symptom, not a disease, and I told him that I could find no physiological defect that would prevent him from performing. I prescribed Viagra and asked him to have sex one or two times a week. Then I spoke with his wife and encouraged her to help him perform and show her desire and interest in him.

When I saw this couple six months later, I was shocked. They both had lost a significant amount of weight, quit drinking, and nearly stopped smoking. They were going to the gym together and had stopped all medications for emotional distress. When I asked the man about sex, he responded confidently, "We are having sex twice a week now, but truly I use Viagra only when the fear of failure comes back."

recognition that they are youthful, sexy, and healthy. Our society maintains different standards of beauty for men and women, so it's especially important for women to feel desired and attractive as they age. Sex plays an important role in that. Women will make a great deal of effort to look sexually attractive to gain the interest, attention, and passion of men.

The other important piece of women's sexuality is the fact that women tend to have all the power in the bedroom. I said this before, but what does it mean? It means that women always decide if sex will happen or not. We know this from watching social interactions between men and women. If a man and woman meet at a bar, who decides if sex is on the table that evening? *The woman does.* The man needs sex; she does not. So she has the power to choose. This ability to turn the sexual faucet on or off can give a woman great power in a relationship—but if it is misused, it can also destroy the relationship.

This is why, in my experience, low libido is such a devastating problem for women and for their relationships if not managed properly. Let's say you're a woman who, for the first forty years of her life, has had a strong libido. You've had a good sex life with your husband and felt desired, feminine, and sexy. But now, after having your last child and maybe moving toward menopause, you find your sex drive diminishing. Now, most of the time, you're uninterested in sex. However, your husband still has his strong libido, so he repeatedly approaches you for sex. But now you find the advances annoying, so you make excuses: you're too tired, you had a hard day. After a while, you either get angry or disengage completely.

If this continues, it becomes more than a problem of different sex drives. You begin to question your identity, your partner's character, and your relationship. Is your husband a sex fiend? Does he think of you only as a vehicle for sex? If you have sex with him when you're not interested, are you letting him exploit you? If this continues, your marriage becomes strained, and you both become distant and angry. Your husband stops approaching you, tired of feeling like he has to "beg" for sex. Does that mean he's less attracted to you, or that you're not sexy anymore? Why can't things just go back to the way they were?

This can quickly spiral downward into the pattern I've seen my entire career. The woman becomes distant and guarded, unwilling to engage in sex without libido. She pushes her husband away, making him the bad guy for wanting sex, but at the same time she feels confused and rejected. The man is angry at his wife because in his mind she is giving up on their marriage. He may cheat to satisfy his sexual needs, or even seek divorce. While all this is happening, nobody is talking. Nobody is consulting the family physician, friends, or anyone else; this important issue will be sitting in a secret box.

So while we continue to look for ways to treat low libido in women, it is vital for women and their husbands to see that the true solution for this problem will come through women adopting a new understanding of their libido and what controls their sex lives.

Low libido in women is *normal*, but women should not let their sexual activity be determined by their libido. "What?" you say. "I have an option here?" Yes! That's what most women don't understand: you can have sexual relations without libido. That isn't an option for men because without libido, there's no erection. But for women, you can choose to have sex without the desire—and you should. In other words, *it's good to have sex even when the desire is not there in the beginning or as strong as it used to be for the moment.*

You don't eat only when you are hungry, but because you need food and it is good for you. You go to the gym in spite of fatigue because you know it's good for you. Women who want to overcome the crisis of low libido should take the same "use it or lose it" attitude toward sex. Sex is good for you. Sex is a gift of nature given to you so you can experience excitement, love, warmth, and happiness. It is rich with many great surprises, so don't let loss of libido rob you of all the other blessings that sex brings to life.

This couple's story illustrates what I mean. The man was forty-six, the woman forty-two. They had two teen kids, but after giving birth to her second child eleven years ago, the woman lost her interest in sexual activity, and gradually she concluded she could do without sex. Life became about the daily routine.

Her husband came to see me for care for anxiety, heart palpitations, and depression. After I questioned him about their sexual activities, he drew a clear picture of their sexual problems. Initially, he made repeated efforts to persuade his wife to have relations with him, but that effort became a humiliating burden because like most men he resented feeling like he needed to beg his wife for sex. He turned to masturbation but grew frustrated and unhappy, and this started to negatively affect his business.

He and his wife basically lived asexual lives, withdrawing gradually from each other. Eventually, she started to wonder whether something was wrong with him, and she asked him to see me. I found no medical problems with the man but a great deal of anxiety and frustration. In our conversation, he told me that he had started having extramarital relations and was planning to divorce his wife. He did not want to break up his family but could not go on with this life without normal sex.

I consulted with his wife, and she admitted losing her libido and surrendering to the idea that life would go on without sex. She never discussed it with her husband nor looked for help from anyone. She thought that if a woman lost her libido, there was nothing that could be done and she and her husband just had to live with it.

I explained sexuality in men and women, the differences between the male and female sexual appetite, and the importance of sex for health and happiness. As she slowly understood what was happening, she paused and then broke into tears. As she regrouped, I asked the reason for her crying. She said. "My husband is a very hard worker, a good family man, and a good father, and I feel I have let him down. Nobody ever told me what you just said, and I was wrong." In that moment, I felt the woman's view of her marriage and herself change.

Fortunately, this story has a happy ending. The woman began to do more to revive her libido and engaged sexually with her husband even when she did not have the desire. Their sexual relations got back to normal, over time she regained a great deal of her libido, and the family stayed united. But many such stories do not end well because no one says anything until it's too late. The husband has an affair or there is a terrible fight, and the marriage breaks up when it could have been saved by an open conversation about sex.

That doesn't have to happen, and much of the power to prevent broken families is in the woman's hands.

SURRENDERING TO LOW LIBIDO RUINS MARRIAGES

ONE OF THE BIGGEST DIFFERENCES I have seen between women and men is that when a man experiences ED or a loss of libido, he might not talk about it, but he will go to the ends of the earth to get his potency back. That's why drugs like Viagra are huge sellers; men want to continue to have sex.

Women are not the same. I have talked with hundreds of women experiencing low libido, and it is common for them to tell me that they are not interested in sex anymore and that this is the way life is. It cannot change, and they are resigned to it. They care about their children and their careers now, and their husbands are just going to have to adapt. "He'll be fine," is a phrase I have heard over and over. No, he won't be fine. While a short-term loss of libido in women is common, a long-term loss of libido in women requires further evaluation. It is often a sign that something else is wrong.

The trouble comes when women *accept* that their libido is gone and there is nothing to be done. It may feel more comfortable not to bother with trying to have sex, just as it is easier not to bother with exercise, but that is not good for the body or soul. Should women take the easy track, surrender their sexuality, and give up such a precious gift with its effect on the motivation to look good and the excitement of living, as well as its important benefits for our immune system? I don't want to see women make that choice.

To choose no sex is to choose the end of marriage. I saw a group of women on television talking about love, marriage, and sex, and one woman stood out. She said, "I am fifty-eight years old. I want a relationship with a man but with no sex. I don't want anything related to sex." The host asked her why, and she said, "I'll tell you the truth. I've had three marriages, and all of them went down the drain, and I don't want to repeat that again." That told me that this woman likely lost her libido, did not address it, and suffered possible consequences in her marriages. She would do better to work with a physician to understand the issue, correct her approach, and understand that maintaining her sexuality is the way to achieve happiness and healthy marital relations.

The tragedy of low libido is that if a woman decides she will live without sex and thinks something is wrong with her husband for wanting sex, her marriage may end up in ashes before she even recognizes that her assumption may be wrong. The problem becomes even worse when a man is dealing with ED because the woman's low libido will only reinforce his feelings of inadequacy. This is the sad progression I see happening again and again:

- The woman finds herself desiring sex less frequently, commonly after menopause, but also after pregnancy and childbirth and sometimes due to other factors ranging from vaginal dryness to feelings of rejection. She may have hot flashes, gain weight, and feel less desirable.

- The man with ED fears that his wife doesn't want to have sex because he doesn't satisfy her. Both partners are locked in their own problems and self-doubts, and *they do not talk about it*. A ten-minute conversation could remedy most of the issues, but instead they each suffer alone with their fears. It is inconceivable that such an important topic that affects our life and happiness is not discussed, but that is quite common.

- Because the man doesn't approach his wife out of fear of rejection, the woman feels like she is no longer desirable.

She stops taking care of herself, gains weight, dresses unattractively, and becomes less attractive to her husband and to herself. This self-hatred can lead to *body dysmorphia*, where the woman perceives herself to have terrible flaws that demand extreme correction, such as cosmetic surgery. At this point, the couple stops the pretense of even trying to have sex.

- Because the man needs sex as men normally do, he finds alternatives. He masturbates, watches porn, or has an affair. The couple descends into resentment, shame, and guilt but still do not communicate about all these troubles. At this point, the marriage is probably beyond saving.

I have seen this happen many times. I had a patient, a man, thirty-eight years old, a father of three, divorced. When I asked him why he was divorced, he told me that his wife had lost her interest in sex after their children were born and rejected his attempts to have sex. He made repeated attempts to pursue her, but she did not want to discuss the issue with him. They had a good relationship, but they were like brother and sister. From her perspective it was a durable, sustainable family unit. Divorce caught her completely by surprise. The wife's libido determined the family's future, and when she listened to that destructive voice telling her that she could live better without sex, she inadvertently tore out the heart of any intimacy, sharing, pleasure, and joy that she and her husband had once enjoyed.

Based on my conversations with many women who have gone through this process, they did not understand the damage that their choice to accept their loss of libido was causing around them until it was too late. Even then they did not understand the strong forces that brought such dramatic changes in their life. They felt that what happened was meant to happen and that they had done their best to prevent it. It is still striking that so many women do not associate their choice to give up sex in their marriage with the eventual destruction of their families. They might blame the trouble on mood swings, weight gain, or infidelity without looking inwardly at their response to their lack of desire for sex. This must change, and it can change.

LOW LIBIDO IS NOT A PRISON

THAT CHANGE STARTS WHEN THE woman decides not to view low libido as something that is "just part of life," something that can never change. It can change, and that begins with a talk with her physician, because low thyroid, diabetes, liver disease, kidney disease, hypertension, and many other medical conditions can all cause low libido. Then, if her health is okay, my female patient and I will talk about lifestyle factors, and there are many.

Some women lose interest in sex because they start to focus on motherhood, which is normal for a period of time. Then, when they settle into parenting and start to feel better about their post-baby body, the sex drive comes back. But women need to take an active role in building libido back to its previous level. Any physiological system that becomes impaired during crisis or trauma needs a period of rehabilitation to restore its capacity. If someone breaks an arm, the arm will require intensive physical therapy and exercise after healing to regain its full use. Sexual capacity and the libido follow the same pattern.

When a woman perceives that she is losing her libido, she might try to find the cause and address it. But if she doesn't put forth effort toward restoring her libido, she may lose her sexuality. Therefore, we need to stress to women that libido will change at times but that long-term loss of libido should be evaluated and addressed medically and emotionally. Abandoning it is a big mistake. Ignorance of the importance of female libido is like a silent epidemic, harming so many women and their families. If a woman doesn't understand her libido, when it drops off or disappears, the most she will do is mention the problem to her ob-gyn and get a pill or hormone cream. Most, however, will accept the libido loss as a permanent fact and try to adapt to it by changing their self-image, their sexual behavior, and their intimate habits. *The blind acceptance of the loss of female libido as the end of jeopardizes happy marriages and families.*

But women are too smart to allow this to go on. With the right guidance and information, they will make better choices. What do I mean?

- First, the female libido can be weak or strong over time, but it never disappears entirely. It can be revived, but the longer you let it atrophy, the harder it will be to bring it back.

- Second, never use libido as a gatekeeper to determine your sexual behavior. It may serve as a catalyst for sexual activity, but libido does not need to be the determining factor in whether or not a woman responds to sexual advances.

- Third, sexuality in women is important to overall physical, mental, and emotional well-being. It should not be surrendered without a fight.

A forty-two-year-old came to my office with her husband having numerous somatic symptoms from head to toe. She had been running to many specialists and taking many medications. She claimed that she lost her libido two years earlier after a hysterectomy, but her ovaries were not removed. She was given hormones including testosterone, but sex was rare, once every one or two months. Her husband was frustrated but loyal and supportive. He had developed some ED due to emotional difficulties with her during intimacy. They were both exhausted, confused, and unhappy but medically healthy. She blamed herself for his ED, and he blamed himself for her loss of libido. I could see that without my intervention, they would not enjoy a good outcome.

I had a long discussion with them explaining the physiology of sexuality. Then I stopped her medications that had a negative effect on the libido. I asked them to exercise together one hour a day and said that, no matter what was blocking them, they should resume sexual activity three times a week.

I saw them again three months later, and I was astonished. Most of the woman's symptoms were gone, she was cheerful and happy, and they were holding hands like teenagers, preparing for a trip to Europe. The man was able to sexually function, using Viagra rarely, and the woman had regained her libido and was achieving orgasm in 50 percent of their sexual encounters.

What a reward from just talk, guidance, and encouragement!

The key to this entire chapter is the idea that for women, sex without libido is not only possible but desirable and should be encouraged. Do it despite of the lack of libido at the time, for your own benefit and needs, to please not only your husband but yourself, for your own sexual pleasure and enjoyment of intimacy.

Women do not need libido to engage in sexual activity. If you start sex, your sexual physiology will take over and create its own momentum to advance into arousal, excitement, orgasm, discharge, and relaxation. Many positive human actions behave in the same way. When we return from work, we may be tired, but we do our exercise routine anyway. Initially it is hard, but soon we feel much better, and when we are done, we feel energetic, strong, and happy. Had we surrendered to the desire to stay on the couch, we would feel lazy and sleepy. As a woman who may be experiencing low libido, say, "I'm going to pursue sex without libido and allow the sexual act itself to stimulate pleasure and satisfaction."

Lack of libido does not mean lack of pleasure. Remember, women derive a great deal of their satisfaction in sex from the closeness and intimacy, not only from arousal and orgasm, though there is nothing that prevents a woman with low libido from experiencing a strong orgasm. In a way, women are much better off than men because if a man's libido goes, he can't get an erection, and he's done with sex. With women, sex is a choice, and she should not deprive herself that choice.

Am I suggesting that women have sex with their partners even when their libido is dormant and they're not feeling sexual desire? *Yes.* I give this advice for the same reason I would advise a person to exercise or brush his teeth: *because it is good for you.* Some women may find that offensive, but doing this is in the woman's best interest. Remember, women have all the sexual power in the relationship, so when she engages with sex, she is exercising that power for her own good and for the good of the relationship. The continuation of successful, satisfying sex creates a *positive* feedback loop in the relationship. The more satisfying sex you have, the more satisfying sex you're going to have, and the better you and your partner will feel about each other and yourselves.

> *Masturbation is one of the best ways for women to get sexual satisfaction and reach orgasm without concerns about ED, rejection, or any other issues, but the topic is still taboo for many women. In a national survey, 21 percent of women said they had never masturbated in their lives, compared with only 8 percent of men.*[4] *But there is nothing perverted or immoral about masturbation, and it is something that all women should be open to if they desire.*

SYMPTOMS AND CAUSES OF LOW LIBIDO

LOSS OF LIBIDO IN WOMEN is not a disease, but a symptom, and like all symptoms, it may be related to many different causes. Low libido is generally the result of a combination of physiological, hormonal, emotional, and psychological factors that affect the female arousal system, which we don't understand very well. There are also various grades of dysfunction: lack of libido, lack of arousal, genital arousal disorder, and orgasmic disorder. There are also a huge range of possible causal factors for low libido, and many of them combine to cause a disinterest in sex:

- menopause

- relationship and life stress

- a negative sexual experience or abuse

- pregnancy

- medications for conditions such as depression, which can cause low libido

- diabetes, cancer, cardiovascular disease, low or high thyroid

- multiple sclerosis or other neurological disorders

- renal, liver, or heart failure

- smoking

- surgery

One surprising finding, however, is that there is no connection between women's testosterone levels and sexual desire. Women produce a small amount of natural testosterone in their bodies, and this does have an effect on libido, but when you give a woman that small amount, it will not have the same effect.[5] Women in menopause who are given estrogen may not respond, either. Hormone therapy is not a quick fix.

However, some of the most common conditions that accompany low libido are seen among women with poor general health, a low education level, depression, anxiety, thyroid conditions, and incontinence.[6] Other factors associated with reduced desire include a partner's sexual dysfunction and infertility, while rewarding factors such as positive past sexual experiences, positive mental health, positive self-image, and high expectations for the relationship are all associated with higher sexual desire in women.[7] Above all, compatibility and a good relationship with her partner will foster a healthy libido.

The conclusion should be clear. When we take away the disappointing results of treating women with testosterone and estrogen, the other factors that most often contribute to low libido are very treatable. Many respond to counseling, lifestyle changes, or greater and more intimate communication between partners. In other words, if women are willing to consider low libido not as a defect or a verdict but as a symptom that can change like other symptoms, huge strides can be made. Just because it's raining one day doesn't mean that tomorrow won't be sunny.

How do you know if you are experiencing low libido? First of all, if you are in premenopause, in menopause, or have already passed through menopause, you are more likely to experience some libido falloff. About half of women at midlife and older experience some kind of sexual dysfunction.[8] This does not mean there's something wrong with you. It means that along with midlife come hormonal changes, relationship changes, and changes to general health that can impact libido. Here are some common signs:

- having no interest in any type of sexual activity, including masturbation

- rarely or never having sexual thoughts or fantasies

- being concerned by your lack of sexual activity or fantasies

- rejecting a partner's sexual overtures

- painful intercourse. Because sex is psychological for women, low libido can cause the vagina to produce less lubrication or have vaginal spasms, making sex uncomfortable.

Experiencing some of these signs does not mean you have a disease or are mishandling your health. It means that you are normal. Emotional factors, a woman's perception of herself and her attractiveness, and the state of the intimate relationship affect libido strongly. It's essential that women understand this and understand that they are not sexually defective or abnormal. Most importantly, because science does not have a clear picture of what causes female low libido or how to treat it, that means that anything you, your spouse, and your doctor can do to treat it is just as valid as the most advanced experimental treatment at the most state-of-the-art hospital. In other words, there are many effective steps you can take.

TREATING LOW LIBIDO

BECAUSE LIBIDO FOR WOMEN IS so connected to trust, affection, and self-esteem, the most effective treatments tend to be the ones that are the least "medical:" talking, sharing, honesty, and trying sex even if libido is not present. However, it is important that we talk about ways to address low libido medically as well:

- **Medication**—Hormone therapy has proven mostly ineffective, but a specialist can offer hormones including progesterone, estrogen, and testosterone administered by cream, pills, or time-released pellets. Some women tell me that it helps them to feel better and improves their libido and the hot flashes. Whether this is the effect of the hormones or the placebo effect, I encourage them to continue as long as they are aware of the risk of cancer and blood clots. The hormones definitely help with hot flashes and sleep, and this can be enough to improve libido.

- Two other medications appear to show some promise for improving female libido. A study confirms that bupropion, a medicine for anxiety and depression, is positive in improving sexual desire, arousal, orgasm completion, and sexual satisfaction.[9] I have been using it for many years, and it does help. The problem is that if I had not been dealing systematically with this topic as a physician on a daily basis, I would probably not have known about this off-label treatment option or known which women to offer it to. Instead of getting relief, they would have continued to suffer along with their partners.

Another medication that offers hope is flibanserin, the first FDA-approved drug for women with low libido. (It is telling that it took thirty years after Viagra was discovered to come up with a sexual drug for women. The researchers were obviously all men.) However, this drug is new and very controversial because of its potential for severe blood-pressure-related side effects, and it needs to be taken daily[10], so I don't use it in my practice. However, it's a good sign that such drugs are being researched, although I believe the best treatment is still open discussion between the partners and the physician. Often, when we let nature take care of us, it will do the best job.

Finally, an injectable drug called bremelanotide was approved recently for use by premenopausal women. But here's the thing about medication: I can't say for certain if it works directly on the libido or reduces emotional stress and thereby indirectly improves libido. The woman's body is not a machine that will respond to pills and injection.

It takes love and tender care to activate her libido. Young women need an understanding and respectful partner who will be compassionate and affectionate. They also need guidance and open dialogue with physicians, friends, and family—and access to informative articles.

This is why I say the libido is like exercise. When you encourage yourself to exercise, you grow to like it, and it becomes something you can't do without. If women give themselves to sex despite their libido, arousal will take its course and lead to excitement, orgasm, and the wonderful feelings that come after. When you do this as a woman, you will be hooked on it! Shots and pills will look easier, but they won't help you in the same way. If you follow my advice, your libido will be flourishing!

- **Counseling**—It makes sense that the emotional and psychological component of female low libido would respond to psychological counseling, and it appears that is the case. One study found that women responded very positively to cognitive-behavioral therapy (CBT), a therapeutic modality that teaches patients to recognize their negative and harmful patterns of thinking and modify them.[11]

I also believe, based on my practice, that couples can benefit from couples counseling with a qualified sex or relationship therapist. Such counseling can help couples break communication logjams, be honest about their sexual needs and fears, and develop better habits to foster intimacy, trust, and respect for each other. This should not be a substitute for a visit with a physician because only your

PCP can rule out physical causes for sexual dysfunction, but a skilled counselor can be a wonderful ally to a caring doctor.

- **Lifestyle changes**—Most of the time, I will recommend that a woman try lifestyle changes as well as communicating with her partner before any more radical treatment. First, *exercise*. There is not a great deal of research looking at the power of specific types of exercise to boost female libido, but we know a few things. Exercise increases energy, improves mood, and with time improves body image, so you feel better about how you look, which is good for sexual desire. There are also a few studies that show that exercise can specifically improve sex drive. One found a positive relationship between physical fitness and sexual health. In other words, the more fit and healthy a person is in general, the better his or her overall sexual functioning.[12] Another study found that yoga improved all markers for sexual function in women, including desire, arousal, lubrication, orgasm, satisfaction, and pain—and the benefits were greater for women over age forty-five![13] Finally, some small studies have shown that Kegel exercises (contractions of the pelvic floor muscles) improve women's overall sexual functioning.[14] In general, exercise is always the right prescription because it benefits everyone in multiple ways.

Another lifestyle change women can make involves *stress*. It's well known how the chemicals that flood the body during chronic episodes of either work-related or relationship stress can wreak havoc, from constricting blood flow to affecting neurotransmitter levels. Stress is proven to affect women's genital arousal—meaning that under high-stress conditions, the clitoris and vagina don't experience the same increases in blood flow and nerve stimulation that lead to arousal and satisfying sex.[15]

The answer, of course, is reducing and managing stress. Try to eliminate the sources of chronic stress from your life. Use exercise and meditation to reduce the effects of stress. Take steps to improve your *sleep*, which can go a long way to reducing the impact of stress. Good sleep is also essential for better health and energy. It may become negatively affected by alcohol or consumption of caffeine, particularly when used in the evening hours.

Finally, women can *change bad habits*. Excessive drinking, smoking, a poor diet—they all damage general health, which, as we've already discussed, negatively affects sexual health. When a woman feels fit, healthy, energetic, beautiful, and confident, she is more likely to be interested in sex. It is pure common sense.

REDRAWING THE UNSPOKEN SEXUAL CONTRACT

HOWEVER, THOSE TREATMENT OPTIONS ARE MINOR compared to the importance of the woman talking with her doctor, talking with her husband, being open about her needs and her fears, and making conscious efforts to engage in sexual activity. Women who choose to break through their low libido and engage in sex, despite having no desire for it at the moment, will often have arousal once they start having sex. Arousal, orgasm, satisfaction—they are all possible even without the initial libido. This is the secret so many women do not know or understand. Sadly, many women stop sex completely when their libido is absent.

In a sense, the issue of choosing sex instead of being a slave to libido is as much about women's rights and equality with men as anything else. Lifelong sex has been seen as something only men should aspire to, but now we're seeing that women have a right to *choose* to be just as sexual as men. This is about the woman being capable and independent to choose the kind of life she wants. Some women might read this and object, saying, "Dr. Kedan is saying that women should service men sexually even when they don't have the desire!" No. That is wrong. No woman should do things just to please a man. Choosing to have sex in the absence of libido is about the *woman's benefit*.

Some women may believe that not engaging in sexual activities when their libido doesn't direct them to do so means they are liberated sexually. But that is the wrong interpretation. If you choose as a woman not to have sex for other reasons, that is a valid choice. But to surrender to the libido when it directs you to give up something as joyous and healthy as sex is to allow an unconscious physiological signal to dictate your happiness, and that can only lead to negative consequences. Choosing to embrace sexuality without letting low libido determine your sexual habits is *freedom* for women.

Since women derive about 80 percent of their satisfaction from sex by sources other than orgasm, they can engage in sex for pleasure by choice, rather than because of a biological drive like men. In other words, when a woman has a low sex drive, she might be perfectly happy, unlike her husband, who is climbing the walls because men *need* sex. Women need sex, too, but its meaning and process are completely different than in men. This is what I am saying:

> *If a woman has low libido but is otherwise healthy, has a loving partner whom she trusts and wants to satisfy, and cares about the health of her relationship, she should consider engaging in sex without the immediate physical desire for it. In my experience, doing so will not only make her partner feel desired and happy, but will also lead to sexual satisfaction for the woman as well as the satisfaction of closeness and intimacy. Furthermore, since regular sex is proven to be good for relationships, sex without libido will increase her happiness by helping her relationship be more engaged, loving, exciting, and romantic. Finally, engaging in sexual activity can actually revive the dormant female libido, so the more sex she has, the more her desire should return.*

Some women will object to this as "being used for sex," but most do not object to the idea once they are in my office, suffering because their marriage is falling apart. They understand once I explain that agreeing to have sex with your husband even when you don't have the desire at that moment is not exploitation. Your man is not exploiting you by coming to you as his life partner for sex, and you are not being objectified by saying yes. You are simply acknowledging the reality that men have a need for sex that women do not possess in the same way. If a woman does not satisfy that need, the man will develop frustration and may look elsewhere for satisfaction. It's that simple. I have seen it over and over again.

So it is in the best interest of both partners if the woman can look at sex as something beneficial for her femininity, her self-esteem, her independence, her pride, and her partner and their relationship. It is time to rewrite that unspoken sexual contract that men and women establish when they get together—a contract that is outdated and damaging. We need to rewrite it according to the line from the Song of Solomon (6:3): "I am my beloved's and my beloved is mine."

There are two polarized social practices that we need to discard. The first says that the woman should obey the man's desire and give him sex at his wish. The second says that the woman should only listen to her own desires and the man is selfish for constantly wanting and needing sex. The second practice says that if the woman's libido diminishes or fails, the man has to say, "Oh well," and accept a sexless marriage.

The alternative and more practical and beneficial approach would be to find harmony between men and women in order to satisfy both partners through respect and mutual understanding of needs. Importantly, women remain in control of their sexual activities. Here is what such an approach might look like:

- As women are in control of their sexual activities, sex is first and foremost for their own enjoyment and benefit. At the same time, however, sexual interaction with her partner is essential for the well-being of her husband and marriage.

- The man must respect that the woman's libido is not like his. It is not revved up all the time, and she does not become aroused instantly. Her sex drive is sensitive to emotional and psychological factors, and he cannot assume it will always be at his service.

- The woman must not treat the man's need for sex as a transaction in which she is "giving him sex," and he is "selfish and demanding." Her attitude should be, "with love and interest, I'm doing my part to keep my dear husband happy and our marriage stronger."

- The woman must never make the man feel as though he is begging for sex. It's humiliating and degrading. She will also never withhold sex as a punishment or tool for persuasion. If she is not happy with the man's behavior, they should sit down and discuss it. There is no room in a healthy relationship for anger and sexual retaliation.

- The man may not keep his fears about his own sexual nonperformance to himself because his wife will see herself as the cause of his nonperformance. Again, communicate.

- The man must understand that women are sensitive to emotional currents and their sexual response is connected to these emotions; therefore he needs to understand and act accordingly. He will make an effort to satisfy the woman's need for postcoital intimacy (in other words, he's not allowed to reach orgasm, turn over, and go to sleep). The Talmud says, "When man reached his orgasm, ending the act, he should remain with his wife to comfort her and show her his sincerity and love so it will not appear like he used her for his own pleasure."

- Both partners will attempt to bring variety and spice into their sex lives.

- Both partners will take care of their bodies. Being overweight or having low energy kills sex drive, harms sexual relations, and makes both men and women feel ashamed of their bodies when they should be celebrating them.

- Both partners will masturbate if they want to without feeling that it is dirty. Masturbation is healthy, natural, and normal.

- The woman will help the man learn to satisfy her sexually in ways that do not involve intercourse. She will guide his hand to her sex organs, use sex toys, and instruct him on how to satisfy her in any way that works for her. This will help her enjoy sex more while helping the man feel more confident that he can satisfy her.

- Both partners will talk openly and regularly about their desires, concerns, and sexual fantasies; it is stimulating and fun, and it opens positive channels so you know you are both on the same page.

This new contract sweeps away all the misperceptions and attitudes about sex that have put so many of my male and female patients in misery and driven many families to break up. It also breaks the news that so many women need to hear:

Having regular sex and enjoying the intimacy and affection that come with it can reawaken the female libido.

This does not always happen, but many of my female patients report wanting sex more and beginning to enjoy sex once they start having it more. I have seen it happen many times, and even women who did not regain most of their sex drive enjoyed arousal and orgasm, felt close to their husbands again, enjoyed feeling desirable, and savored the intimacy, play, and pleasure of sex. I have seen many marriages saved because women had the courage and caring to set aside their old attitudes about libido and choose to have sex for pleasure.

It is ironic that a simple act of reeducating men and women about the role of libido and relationships could repair many of the broken marriages, fractured families, and lonely, displaced children in our society. Instead of relying on medication and surgery, the solution turns out to be communication, understanding, and love! Amazing.

SEX IS AN ABSOLUTE GOOD

SEX, SIMPLY PUT, IS AN ESSENTIAL part of a strong relationship. It is difficult, if not impossible, to have a strong, lasting relationship without it. That is why I say that for women, sex is like exercise: it is good for you even if you don't feel like doing it at that moment. It is also good for your man and for your marriage. Letting go of the old attitudes about libido will allow women to see that sex really is an absolute good in their marriages, a benefit to their self-image, confidence, drive, and life.

If a woman surrenders to low libido and declines to have sex, she may lose the incentive to take care of herself and maintain her appearance, health, good diet, exercise program, and more. Meanwhile, because the man's sex drive continues unabated, he will be motivated to stay fit and look good, but if his wife has given up on sex due to low libido, his sexual energy may be channeled toward some other woman, or he may become frustrated, unsatisfied, and unhappy. I always tell my patients that happiness and depression are contagious, so your husband's mood may infect your entire home and life.

On the other hand, if a woman keeps sex in her marriage despite the ups and downs of her libido, she will continue to feel desired and satisfied. Her confidence and self-esteem will be strong. Her husband will desire her. She'll be motivated to work out, eat right, dress well, quit bad habits, and be sexy. Her husband will do the same. Caring about sex and intimacy becomes its own virtuous cycle.

So when the choice lies before you as a woman, choose sex when it's possible, even if your libido is low. You will end up enjoying the process—being loved and loving your beloved, and you will feel vital and young and close and naughty and playful and delightfully exhausted. I have seen it among young as well as old couples, and those couples never age in their spirit or in their affection.

If you're in menopause and your vagina is dry, use lubricating jelly. If your husband has ED, guide him to stimulate you in other ways and help him overcome the fear of performance difficulties by talking to your doctor. Be patient, open, understanding, and loving. This is correctable. Learn each other's positive and negative points, enhance the positive, and correct or bypass the negative.

Some time ago, I was treating a forty-four-year-old woman, married sixteen years to her forty-two-year-old husband. No kids. The sex had been good, and they were both healthy. Six years earlier, she had a hysterectomy and lost her desire for sex, but she still had her ovaries, so her body was still producing estrogen. However, for those six years, she had not allowed her husband to touch her. When she came to see me, she told me he was frustrated, angry, masturbating, and unhappy. They were not talking to each other or trying to understand the problem.

The woman was confused, depressed, and had probably gone into menopause as well. But she was bewildered about her loss of libido. She had already decided she was inadequate and decided that something was medically wrong with her. When you tell yourself that you're sick, you can experience symptoms of low energy and depression and can even develop physical disorders like high blood pressure, ulcers, or thyroid disease. She had started to gain weight and lose her energy and stamina, and she had no motivation to feel attractive or feminine.

Her loss of libido was the source of the problem, but she didn't realize it. She said, "I'm depressed; I'm unhappy; I'm sick; something's wrong with me." But I indicated to her that in fact, until her surgery, she had been fine. I told her that she was healthy. She told me that she had never talked to anyone about how she was feeling, including the person she should have talked to first—her husband. That is a terrible burden to carry, holding fear and guilt alone, without support.

All I did was open her mind to this new way to think about her libido and sexuality in her marriage. This is why I say I learn more medicine from my patients than I did from my teachers. We discussed all this, and she agreed to start over again. I explained her libido in detail and asked her to attempt to have sexual activity with her husband on a regular basis no matter what her desire was like in the moment. I asked her to exercise daily and return to see me in four months. She left my office excited, happier, and armed with encouragement and direction. Suddenly, she didn't feel powerless and weak any longer.

Four months later, she came to see me again. Now, she was happy. She and her husband were having sex twice a week. She reached orgasm infrequently, but she didn't care. She was enjoying the closeness and the intimacy, and best of all her libido had started to improve! As the Israelis say, "Don't worry if you have no appetite, just eat, and the appetite comes with the eating." All I did was talk to her and show her the path. I didn't give her a pill or hormone therapy. I helped her think differently. Now she was happy and healthy again, and her marriage had significantly improved.

This is why I want more women with low libido to treat sex like exercise—as something beneficial that will make them feel great, even if they don't want to do it. Even if you get up one morning and say, "I'm sore; I just want to go back to bed. I don't want to go to the gym," but you do it anyway. You never regret it. Number one, exercise is very good for you. Number two, after you are done, you say, "That felt great! I'm so glad I did this." Sex works the same way.

Don't surrender to low libido. Sexual activity is important and determines the future of the relationship and the family. If women make a conscious effort to have sex despite low libido, not only will they get enjoyment from it, but their libido will often improve. If your man has dysfunction, work in concert with him and his doctor to help him regain his confidence and remove fear, while working with your doctor to address your own low libido.

Doing all this shows that you care about your marriage and your partner and that can go a long way to helping you both enjoy work, leisure, family, and everything else in life. Look at life as a game, play it with all the tools available to you, and have fun. Sex is nature's gift to us, and it can be available for you throughout your life if you appreciate it and use it.

Chapter Six

COMMUNICATION IS THE **KEY**

Patients come to me expecting me to have all the answers. That is unrealistic. Physicians should be humble about what we don't know and just as humble about the fact that sometimes the cure for a problem may have nothing to do directly with a pill, a shot, or a surgical procedure.

Sometimes, patients come to me saying that a doctor has given their friend or relative a few months to live, and I reply, "Please don't take them seriously. All they can do is predict based on statistics." I have seen cases where the patient was supposed to be dead but came back to life and lived to collect Social Security. The human body is a marvelous, unpredictable thing, and doctors don't know everything.

When a man comes into my office for sexual dysfunction, he usually comes for another medical issue like high blood pressure. After I ask him about his sexuality, I tell him about the three systems that have to work together—hormonal, circulatory, and nervous—in order for his sexual system to function. I will look for signs and symptoms indicating that these systems are not working as they should be—test his blood glucose, do an ultrasound of his blood vessels, run tests of his liver and kidneys, and so on. Then, if nothing is wrong and all systems are functioning as they should, I'll explain that he's fine and there is nothing physiologically wrong with him that would explain his ED.

Then he'll look frustrated and puzzled and ask me why he's having this problem, and I'll say, "Because your head has to give the order. Your problem is there, so that's what we're going to fix."

Many of the problems and pain I see are due to a crisis of intimacy—men and women wrapped up in their own embarrassment, sure that the other person won't understand or will laugh at them. So they don't share their fear and uncertainty. But secrecy is destructive. For men, it destroys their confidence because they are afraid their wives won't understand, and they develop performance anxiety trying to conceal their "defect" from the spouse. Imagine someone who is a wonderful piano player . . . as long as he is playing in the privacy of his home. Then I tell him, "I'm bringing an audience of people to see you." He falls apart and cannot play from fear of failure. That's what happens to these men.

Women respond differently. When they fear their husband will not understand their low libido, they retreat and grow cold, shut off, and refuse to talk about sex. The man will be perplexed, frequently telling me, "She will not talk; she just declines sex and moves on." They may project the blame on the man, saying that he is at fault for requesting sex or that he is preoccupied with sex or dirty thoughts. They become asexual and treat anything related to sex as negative and wrong.

What I found by inquiry of these women is that they really don't have an answer. All they know is that their sexual desire is not there, so they believe they need to decline sex. Since they have no explanation to give to their husbands, they say nothing. But inside them is a world of thoughts and feelings, and I discover that my talking to them helps them be more open and comfortable talking about their sexual problems.

As a result, I have insight into the thinking of most of the women who struggle with lack of libido. Very few will take the initiative to go to their gynecologist to ask for advice. They really think that something must be wrong with them that caused them to lose their libido, and they surrender to this unknown by giving up their sexuality. By being silent, they can avoid exposure, confrontation, embarrassment, and guilt.

When a man develops the perception that he is sexually inadequate, it will feel like a defeat. He will experience paralysis and shame, which will have serious effects on his motivation and self-respect. Therefore, the usual reaction is to conceal this "defect" by making excuses and avoiding sexual interaction. And so, like the woman, he becomes silent. Now we have both woman and man living in silence. No intimacy or love can happen in such a situation.

In life, we all develop various difficulties and issues and to deal with them, we look for understanding and solutions. We might do an internet search, consult with experts, or talk to family and friends. But sex remains the one taboo topic, the one we do not talk about openly. Therefore, men and women struggling with sexual difficulties tend to live in secrecy and shame.

However, when a husband and wife are encouraged to talk openly to each other—and when their physician helps them feel safe in talking by assuring them that nothing is wrong with them—they are always surprised at how receptive, how understanding, and how relieved the other person is that the silence is broken. Both are always grateful they are being given the chance to make things better by direct communication.

I had a female patient who went through all this with her husband over his ED. After she finally spoke to her husband about it and he told her about the agony he was going through, she felt his pain and acknowledged that avoiding talking to her husband made his suffering worse. She met with me and broke into tears. I asked her why she was crying, and she said, "Because I feel guilty that I ignored my husband's needs." She had no idea that he was suffering.

Communication is the solution to most of the sexual problems that I see. Even if the man needs Viagra, if he and the woman would simply talk, listen, be honest, and break the secrecy and shame surrounding their dysfunction, a lot of marriages would be saved, and many couples would become happier.

Based on my years of observing patients, I would say that 80 percent of the people I see are affected by some sort of sexual dysfunction, theirs or their partners'. All are happy to finally have the opportunity to talk to a professional about it. What surprises me most is that until I opened the conversation with them, they did not recognize that they had a problem, like the couple in their fifties who stopped sex five years before just because they were too busy or the lady who granted her husband sex once a month and no more. As people don't discuss this with anybody because of the taboos, they believe there is something wrong with them.

They believe this is a problem that can't be solved. They believe they are alone and no one will understand.

The first step is to train people to talk to their doctor. The second step is to get them talking to each other. The rest will take care of itself.

BETTER COMMUNICATION = BETTER SEX

RESEARCHERS HAVE FOUND that we don't talk with each other about sex for a variety of reasons: embarrassment, fear the other person will find out about our lack of experience or maybe our fantasies, or the belief that sex comes naturally and we shouldn't have to talk about it. However, many studies have found that sexual communication between couples is linked to greater relationship closeness, higher levels of sexual and relationship satisfaction, more intimacy, and higher levels of birth-control use.[1]

In my years of practice, I have seen the same pattern: one or both partners won't talk about their problems with sex and tell me that they "can't talk to the other person." Why? Because they are afraid of being judged, feeling ashamed, or being rejected. There is also the terrible assumption that bad sex is "just something you have to live with." Then when I finally convince the man or woman to open a dialogue with the other partner about what's been going on, the results are miraculous. Not only can trust be restored, but the man and the woman learn things about each other that they never knew, even after twenty-five years of marriage. Healing starts and sex resumes.

Colorado-based couples therapist Susan Heitler backs this up. She writes:

A great relationship also means good communication in the sense that when differences arise, the partners can talk through their dilemma cooperatively. Differences don't become barriers—they become opportunities to find win-win understandings and solutions.

Making decisions together in a win-win way requires strong collaborative communication skills. Both partners need to be able to talk in a way that when they say things, their partner wants to listen—and when their partner says things, they want to hear them.

Strong communication skills enable couples not only to have fun and share their love, but also to deal with the difficult issues they inevitably will face as they proceed as partners in the business of living.[2]

Interestingly, the value of sexual communication in a relationship is different for men and women. One study[3] found this:

Specifically, we found support for the idea that open sexual communication relates to overall relationship satisfaction differently in men and women as a function of the length of the relationship. For males, open sexual communication was more important for relationship satisfaction at the start of a relationship, and less important as the relationship progresses beyond one year's duration. In contrast, for women in our sample, open sexual communication was more important for relationship satisfaction when the relationship was over one year old, and less important for relationships of less than one year's duration.

That finding highlights the importance of both partners adapting to each other's communication needs as the relationship goes on. Because communication is more important to women as time goes by, men may need to make an effort to communicate more openly and regularly with their wives to keep things intimate and healthy. And because communication is important to men as the relationship progresses, it is important for women to watch for signs that there is a problem the man won't talk about and find ways of opening a discussion about them. Women often have the capability to adapt and improvise solutions better than men do, but they cannot use this ability when they are kept in the dark. The more they learn about their partner, the more they can help with his sexual issues.

DON'T MAKE LIBIDO THE GATEKEEPER

AS WE DISCUSSED EARLIER, one of the barriers to communication is the misunderstanding that both men and women have about the role of sex. Many women feel that they are expected to have sex with their men even when they have no interest in it—to "put out," to use a vulgar common term. In years of observing and speaking with female patients and helping them address sexual concerns, many women have told me that they felt like having sex with their husbands even when their libido is low is their "responsibility." This makes some women feel disrespected and even objectified.

I understand, but those feelings do not change the reality that the male sex drive is much stronger than the female sex drive. Men *need* sex. The surge of testosterone coursing through the veins of every man demands release, and when men cannot release the energy, aggression, and competitive instinct that comes with that hormone, they will eventually turn to negative outlets like rage and violence. Some women claim that the male urge needs to be tamed and controlled, as men are not expected to act like animals in a civilized world, but society has to follow the rules of nature. Yes, men should not act like rampaging beasts, but believing that we can "tame" the male sex drive is not sustainable.

So while women might not like the idea that they ought to have sex with their husbands even when the drive is not there, the simple truth is that *having sex with your husband is the best thing you can do for yourself, your quality of life, and your marriage.* Wrong interpretations, like "You are giving your body to be used by your husband," are part of the problem and distort the role of human sexuality, which is based on love, unity, and devotion.

The attitude that women should only have sex when their libido is strong and that withholding sex is normal and something their man just has to "understand" comes from a time when science did not know that women normally experience lower libido and can do so at any age. Now we know that changes in libido are something that many, if not most, women will experience. Because of this, our understanding of the sexual agreement between man and woman must change, be clarified, and be followed.

It is all right for women to have sex simply for the well-being of the relationship. Sexual activity brings tremendous benefits to a woman's confidence, health, and sense of well-being.

There's no exploitation in this. This is the woman exercising control and making a wise choice to do what is best for both partners. You as the woman have all the control here. Sex is an essential part of a healthy relationship, not a one-sided luxury, and by making the choice to engage in sex despite your low libido, you make the right move for yourself and your spouse. Based on long years of observing couples who have done this, I know the results are consistently positive:

- Libido frequently improves for the woman.

- Happiness and confidence increase.

- Upon beginning sex, she becomes physiologically aroused and frequently reaches orgasm.

- The couple becomes more intimate and closer, with more positive signs like sexual teasing, romantic evenings, and paying greater attention to fitness, grooming, and looking better.

The last one is the real payoff for the woman because women and men get pleasure from sex differently. For men, it is all about the orgasm. A woman can be satisfied by reaching orgasm but can also get a rich reward from feeling feminine and attractive and being close and loved. Sex for a woman is like a diamond necklace: she will enjoy it most when she wears it.

Women should not make sexual decisions based only on libido because it will fool you. Instead, take charge and do what you know is good for your relationship, which will be good for you as well. Make the decision based on its benefit in the same way you make decisions to exercise or eat a healthy diet. Sex is great for your physical and mental health, and if it is loving and giving while you are both healthy, once you become aroused, the sex will be enjoyable and fulfilling. You will demonstrate to yourself that you are beloved and desired, and you will prove to yourself that you are in control of your sexuality.

With that in mind, please know that I am not suggesting that you agree to sex with a man who is demanding, verbally abusive, or physically abusive. You are no one's sexual slave. If your relationship is that damaged, it is not your responsibility to save it through sex.

This is one example of the practical power of the libido. The man is fifty-six, a police officer ready to retire from service in one year. His wife is fifty-two, and they have been married for twenty-eight years. They are grandparents. The wife is happy and busy with her grandchildren, and over the last five years, her sexual response to her husband has dwindled down to nothing. He grew frustrated because she would not even discuss sex with him, and I treated him for insomnia, abdominal cramps, and other somatic symptoms related to his sexual frustration.

As he got closer to retirement, the man was planning to purchase a recreational vehicle and travel all over the country, then buy a summer home. Now he told me that he had put everything on hold and was rethinking his marriage. I decided to discuss the issue with his wife—a charming lady. When it came to sex, she said that she had lost her libido and had no interest. When I asked her about her husband's sexual needs, her response suggested it wasn't something she should bother with. As intelligent as she was, I wondered how she could believe that her husband's sexual happiness had nothing to do with her. Sadly, I have seen this often. I frequently find that women are lacking guidance on the basics of sexuality.

I talked at length with this lady about the differences between male and female sexuality; she did not have the first clue about any of it. She had assumed that because she didn't have the desire for sex, it was perfectly fine to eliminate sex from her married life and no one would suffer any negative consequences.

Six months later I again saw the husband, and the first thing he showed me was a photo on his phone of his big camper and a photo of the little summer house he and his wife had bought. He said he would retire in six months, and they would drive across the country. He did not mention any of his somatic symptoms nor the sexual issue that was the true problem. I asked about sex, and he said that the pills that I gave to his wife worked well and she was back to her regular sexual behavior, like the old days.

I never gave his wife a pill of any kind. No surgery was done, and no specialist was called. All it took was fifteen minutes of teaching and conversation that should have been done back when this lady was in high school. Sex lives forever, and it will come back no matter what you do to it. The only thing that can kill sexuality is ignorance.

SEXUAL DYSFUNCTION AS A REFLECTION OF LOSS OF CONFIDENCE AND POOR COMMUNICATION

A woman, forty-two, noticed that her husband, fifty-two, was showing negative behavioral changes that caused her to lose sleep and experience abdominal cramps, diarrhea, and heart palpitations. She noticed that his personality had changed; he had lost his confidence as a successful businessman and was frequently angry and fearful that he would fail. He became frightened about the future and lost his drive. She also noticed that he lost his interest in sex and over the last five months had avoided approaching her. She asked me to see him to find out what was wrong with him.

The man came in for a physical a week later. He complained of fatigue, weakness, muscle spasms, and dizziness, but mentioned nothing about sex. When I inquired about his sex life, he told me that he thought he was suffering from some kind of physical illness that caused him to be impotent. He would not engage in sexual activity to avoid disappointing his wife and embarrassing himself.

My cooperation with his wife and our open discussion made it easier for me to progress toward a resolution. After running the pertinent tests, I came to the conclusion that he was healthy. However, because of the stress in his business, he failed to perform sexually and eventually developed the terrifying belief that he had become impotent for life. We discussed this, and with reassurances from me along with his wife's participation, the problem eased, and they were able to return to a normal, healthy sex life.

It was shocking and dramatic to see how something a man harbored on his mind could drastically alter his behavior and personality, affect his career, destroy his sexual performance, and nearly ruin his marital life. But it was equally shocking to see how simple and easy the problem was to resolve just by breaking the taboo and ending the secrecy.

MEN, BE REASONABLE AND UNDERSTANDING

NONE OF THIS MEANS THAT men have a free pass to demand sex from their wives at any time. There is nothing primitive or animalistic about needing sex, so long as you treat your partner's pleasure as just as important as your own. Your wife agreeing to sex without libido is an act of generosity and wisdom, and that means that you should do everything you can do ensure that she enjoys sexual satisfaction as much as you do.

If you are callous or rude, if you expect your wife to drop everything to service your needs, or if you insist on having sex when she's exhausted or not feeling well, then you deserve her anger and rejection. Just as I am asking women to make a choice that serves the long-term well-being of their relationship, I am asking men to appreciate that when your woman agrees to sex when she does not feel the desire, she is doing something exceptionally generous and loving. She is not "doing you a favor."

But sex should not feel like a transaction. It should not be, "Honey, if we have sex, I'll mow the lawn." That is crass and exploitative. But you should also not feel like your wife is submitting to you reluctantly. When that happens, men feel like they are begging for sex, and nothing is more humiliating to a man than feeling like he has to beg his wife for sex.

The solution is communication. Husband and wife should sit down and have an honest discussion about the ground rules surrounding sex in their relationship. The man should be clear that he loves his wife, that his sex drive is strong, and that he wants to be with her and satisfy her. The woman should be clear that she loves her husband, finds him attractive, and is happy to have sex as an act of love, intimacy, and mutual pleasure. There should be an understanding that attending to the man's need for sex is a privilege of living in partnership, part of the love and care of each other's needs. I am not suggesting that this is a "wifely duty," but simply a reality of long-term relationships that women must acknowledge . . . and men must respect.

Finally, this does not mean that you as a woman must have sex with your husband every time he asks for it. If you are busy, tired, not feeling well, or emotionally upset, it is perfectly fine to tell him no. But please communicate—take the time to explain why, and don't give him the cold shoulder and make him feel he is not wanted. Be sure your husband understands that you are not cutting him off from sex, punishing him, or beginning some period of no sex that might fill him with dread and loneliness. At the heart of this arrangement is mutual respect: respect for the man's needs and the woman's awareness and respect for the sanctity and health of your relationship that will only be enhanced by regular sex.

As psychologist Harriet Lerner, PhD, writes:

> *If your partner is a good person, and a responsible citizen in the relationship, pushing yourself to have sex once in a while can keep your libido from going into deep freeze especially if children come along. There is often at least one person in a couple who will not feel a "natural urge" to initiate sex but may be able to get into it when they really try. If you're not aroused, there's still something to be said for doing something for your partner's pleasure, and being open to simply enjoying the physical closeness.[4]*

The Facts on Aphrodisiacs

For as long as there have been men and women, there have been claims that eating or drinking this or that would stimulate desire, improve potency, improve fertility, lead to better sexual performance, and improve orgasm. But while there are some botanicals like Chlorophytum borivilianum and Panax ginseng that show promise in laboratory testing, research has found that most of the commercial products on the market that promise sexual benefits are useless and in some cases, potentially harmful.[5] If you feel the need for something to stimulate desire and potency, talk to your physician. Or simply try one of the proven ways to get the sexual fires burning: a good workout and intimate conversation.

COMMUNICATE WITH YOUR PHYSICIAN, TOO

THE OTHER PERSON YOU AND your spouse should be communicating with when dealing with sexual dysfunction or a lack of sex is your personal physician. The first reason is simple: it's important to rule out physiological reasons for ED or a female low libido, which could be something as simple as a medication that affects desire. The right doctor can assess your situation and identify potential medical causes for some sexual problems. That takes away some of the guilt because both partners know they are not choosing to have sexual problems.

If everything is fine physiologically, then your doctor can be an objective third party who can help you figure out the psychological and emotional reasons behind your sexual problems. He or she can explain to you how the male and female sexual systems work, how desire differs for the two genders, and how you may be able to manage those differences. Your physician may also be able to suggest measures to get the fire back in your sex life, from Viagra to working out together to counseling.

Of course, you may not be lucky enough to have a physician who is willing to talk about your sexual issues as anything more than a part of your physical functioning. That's a problem; many medical school graduates are ill-equipped to talk about sex and are uncomfortable doing so. If that's your situation, I suggest that you look for a new physician and take the time to find someone who is willing to talk with you and experienced in addressing sexual problems with candor, patience, and compassion.

HUMILITY, HUMOR, AND SELF-AWARENESS

THIS CHAPTER SHOULD MAKE IT clear that there is hope for a couple experiencing stress, anger, health problems, and fear of divorce due to sexual issues. But that hope only comes when you break your silence and communicate.

Women, please talk to your husbands. Listen and understand their needs; they have a lot to say that you don't know or understand as woman. Men, do the same. Tell your wife your problems and explain your needs, and then listen to hers. Come up with a plan together to accomplish the best results. Keeping quiet to avoid shame or because you think the other person "won't understand" will only lead to disaster.

I see couples get past this hurdle by talking and being committed to changing the rules of their relationship. But I see just as many for whom it is too late—who have waited until the wounds are too deep, there has been infidelity, or things have been said that can't be taken back. It takes humility, generosity, and self-awareness to be willing to listen, admit your role in the problems, be flexible, and put your mutual well-being first. But you can do it. Here are some of my best recommendations:

- Stop judging each other. Don't attach blame for anything. Everyone is trying to do the best they can.

- Talk openly about your problems, fears, failures, and even your sexual fantasies. Maintain a sense of humor and a sense of adventure. Tell your spouse what brings you pleasure because what brings your spouse pleasure might be quite different.

- Make time for each other. No one wants to feel like an afterthought or an intrusion.

- If your problems need a referee or there are bigger issues like infidelity, seek the help of a couples counselor with experience dealing with sexual issues.

- Schedule sex like you would schedule anything else therapeutic: a massage, yoga, therapy, a session in a float tank.

- If having sex when one partner has low libido seems awkward, work hard to stimulate your partner the way he or she likes. Think about it as relationship therapy. Eventually, as you enjoy it, it will become something more.

- Be patient. This will take time.

- Continue communicating regularly about what's happening and how you're feeling. Talk, share, and be transparent. Ask your partner what he or she enjoys in bed and what your partner wants to try. Talk about your emotions. Have fun together. Be adventurous. The more you learn about your partner, the better you can please and accommodate him or her. Show interest in doing that by sharing secrets and feelings.

This really does work. Here is an example. I had a female patient, forty-four with two children, eleven and thirteen. After becoming a mother, she lost interest in sex. Her husband became humiliated and frustrated at her rejection and hated the idea that he had to beg her for sex. Over the years, he began avoiding asking for sex and courting because it became too much effort and seemed humiliating. He would have to ask ten or twenty times over two months to have sex once or twice. He gave up and started to masturbate.

His wife started to ask why he wasn't interested in sex. The situation became clear: she liked having him come to her and beg for sex. It gave her a feeling of control and power. It was flattering. But she had no idea what she was doing. She actually tried to send him to me for a physical to find out what was wrong with *him*! She was denying responsibility, and she had never talked to him about her lack of sexual desire.

The husband did come to see me, and when I asked him about his sex life (I couldn't share with him what his wife had told me because of patient confidentiality), he said that his marriage had been unhappy for several years. "We are not happy, we are not communicating, and I'm sick and tired of begging for sex." He was a successful businessman and very confident, and he had come to resent his wife. They had grown apart. He acknowledged that she was a wonderful woman, a good mother, the usual things I hear. But he could not continue like this, and he was planning to leave his wife and have an extramarital relationship. It was very sad.

They had not talked about any of this. How could either of them expect to know what the other was suffering? What would this do to their family? I asked them to open up and talk about what they both wanted and needed and told them that this might help save their marriage. I saw them four months later as a couple, and they were still married and seeing a sex therapist, and it looked like they might be able to repair their relationship.

The moral of the story? Communicate. It will not fix every sexual problem and every relationship, but no healing can begin until you talk to each other.

Here's one final story for this chapter about a couple who taught me a great deal. He is fifty-two, an engineer, and married for twenty-five years to a woman, forty-eight. They have three kids, one in college, the other two in high school. The woman is devoted to the kids and to her duty as a housewife. He is a devoted father who is active with the kids and works in the yard. But things started to change between them during the past five years when she started declining sexual activity, always telling him that she was too tired or too busy.

He tried hard to convince her to have sex but gave up because he felt insulted. They continued their family activities, were cordial to each other, and showed up for social activities. It appeared that nothing had changed. However, their intimate life, closeness, affection, and warmth were gone, replaced by silence. They were like brother and sister. The woman was making long-term plans for when they would retire and take international trips and cruises and have fun.

Meanwhile, the man's sexual tension and anger grew. First, he relieved it by masturbation. Then he was charmed by one of his secretaries and started an affair with her. As that extramarital relationship became closer, he told me that as much as he cares about his wife and his family, he sees no future in this marriage. Therefore, he decided to divorce his wife and marry his lover. When he broke the news to his wife, she was shocked.

After she regrouped, she came to me, broken, frightened, and in disarray. She kept repeating, "I don't understand. It makes no sense to me, why he is doing this to me and to the kids. What happened to him?" I comforted her with encouragement to keep taking care of herself and the kids, but there wasn't anything else I could do. The experience was difficult for him but devastating for her.

Can we learn a lesson from this couple and from the numerous other couples I have seen in my practice? Yes. Please talk to each other and show each other love and consideration. Do not assume the other person knows what you are feeling or knows what is at stake. Communicate. Silence will only get you heartache.

Chapter Seven

SEXUAL HEALTH EQUALS TOTAL WELL-BEING

One of the premises of this book is that sexual health equals overall health. I think this story illustrates very well how the two interrelate. One of the things I see commonly is depression among people having sexual problems. I had a patient, a forty-six-year-old female, who was obese. She and her husband had not had sex in six years, and she had gained sixty pounds in that time.

After she had been my patient for some time, I saw her husband, age forty-eight, and he was also obese. They were both afraid to have sex because of shame. Their body image was very poor, and they were ashamed of being in that condition. They felt fat and ugly, and they had no energy. They had no interest in engaging in positive things like exercise. The only mutual interest they shared was cooking and eating. As a result, they both continued to gain weight and slid deeper into unhappiness and depression. They had insomnia and were taking sleeping pills, and the woman was having hot flashes. However, they both were intelligent, smart, and cooperative. They were looking for way out of their trap and needed only direction.

I examined them and when we had our consultation, I said I wanted them to exercise at least five hours a week and do many of those hours together. I told them to count calories for each other, eat nothing between the meals, and eat no more than twelve hundred calories per day. Finally, I asked them to start sexual activity in any way they could, even manually, and do it one to three times a week. They agreed to try.

Six months later, I saw the woman, who had obviously lost weight. I asked, "How is your sexual activity?" She perked up and became happy and proud. She told me she had lost twenty pounds and her husband had lost thirty. They were exercising daily and doing many things together besides cooking. They were not taking sleeping pills or anything for depression. They were having sex once or twice a week at least. Sometimes she had to help him ejaculate manually because he had issues keeping an erection, but he did the same for her, and they were learning about each other's bodies and feeling satisfied. I knew that if they continued, they would both lose a lot more weight, their libido would improve, and the man's ED would probably be cured because his circulatory system would become healthier. Their lives would be completely changed.

THE CHICKEN AND THE EGG

SO, WHICH IS IT? Does more healthy sex lead to better overall health, or does being healthier in general lead to better sex? The answer is both. Along with exercise, a healthy diet, sleep, and perhaps meditation, good sex is one of the activities that has virtually no downsides for your well-being. Think of sex and health as a sort of "virtuous cycle": if you have more sex, you are likely to feel better about yourself, sleep better, and have a more positive mood. In turn, that will lead you to want to look better, which leads to exercise, more energy, and a healthy diet, which makes you want to have more sex! How can you go wrong?

Science and my experience as a physician both show that sexual health is not a luxury. It is a vital component of individual well-being. If we treat health holistically, caring for the whole person instead of a collection of systems and symptoms, then we must look at sex as an essential part of overall well-being.

For example, when a person loses his appetite and stops eating, we wonder what's wrong with him. We search the etiology, first by taking a complete and detailed medical history. Next, we do specific tests to find out if one system or another is failing: his gastrointestinal system, his endocrine system, and so on. But what if the tests show that all those systems are fine? Too many physicians then dismiss the problem as being "all in the patient's head" because they can't find a physiological cause. But problems with the head—sadness, stress, frustration, shame—are just as real and just as important as problems with the heart, lungs, or brain. Good physicians must treat those problems because we are about caring for the whole person, not just a group of systems.

Physicians must be careful not to lose themselves in tests and differential diagnoses and fail the commonsense test. A patient may lose sexual drive for one of many reasons, but he or she will rarely go to the doctor and complain. A sexual problem is considered secret, private, and too personal to be discussed. But how can we expect a layperson to understand the problem and how it can be treated if they feel the person can't discuss it with a professional? This is where the physician has to consider the whole person and where the patient has to ignore society's taboos and be brave enough to speak up.

Here is one example: a male patient, forty-eight years old and married for sixteen years, was recently divorced because three years prior he developed ED. He was so ashamed and humiliated that he decided to divorce and live alone in his apartment. That is like putting yourself in prison!

He came to me for blood pressure and depression that his previous physician had treated with two medications. When I asked my usual questions about his sexual activity, he said he wanted nothing to do with women but was masturbating.

This sounded odd, and after I pressed, he admitted that he had never told any doctor about his ED because of embarrassment and shame. Tests confirmed he was a healthy man, but in reviewing his medications, it was obvious that both medications had similar side effects: they could reduce libido *and* cause ED. It was simple to change both to medications that were just as effective with no sexual side effects.

Three months later, the patient came back for a follow-up. He surprised me with his happy mood and said that he had gotten back together with his wife. He felt the courage to return to normal sexual activities one to two times time a week, and they were very happy together. His children knew nothing about all this but were happy that their mom and dad were back together. Before leaving the office, he handed me his bottle of depression pills and said, "Thank you, Doc, I don't need it anymore!"

Please don't allow fear, embarrassment, or the old-fashioned rules of society to keep you from discussing your intimate problems with your spouse and your doctor. You have nothing to lose and everything to gain.

YES, SEX IS GOOD FOR YOU

AS I HAVE ALREADY SAID, there is a great deal of research showing that sex is good for our general health and well-being. Here is a marvelous perspective on sexual health from the Centers for Disease Control and Prevention (CDC)/Health Resources and Services Administration Advisory Committee on HIV, Viral Hepatitis, and STD Prevention and Treatment (CHAC):

> *Sexual health is a state of well-being in relation to sexuality across the life span that involves physical, emotional, mental, social, and spiritual dimensions. Sexual health is an intrinsic element of human health and is based on a positive, equitable, and respectful approach to sexuality, relationships, and reproduction, that is free of coercion, fear, discrimination, stigma, shame, and violence. It includes: the ability to understand the benefits, risks, and responsibilities of sexual behavior; the prevention and care of disease and other adverse outcomes; and the possibility*

of fulfilling sexual relationships. Sexual health is impacted by socioeconomic and cultural contexts—including policies, practices, and services—that support healthy outcomes for individuals, families, and their communities.[1]

I could not agree with that statement more. There is also additional evidence that sex leads to improved outcomes in a wide range of health areas, including:

- **Better immune function**—Research shows that frequent sex increases the body's levels of an antibody that's important for the immune system.[2] So having more good sex could keep you from catching a cold! Through many years of practice and questioning my patients about their sexual activity, it has become clear that those with active sex lives, no matter their age, always appear to be more vital and healthier, happy and confident in themselves and the future. Be like those people!

- **Improved migraines**—A German study[3] found that 60 percent of people suffering from migraines (which affect women more than men) reported less pain after engaging in sex. Considering the misery that migraines bring, that is significant.

- **Lower heart disease risk**—A study that looked at men in their fifties found that men who have sex at least twice per week have a 45 percent lower risk of heart disease than men who have sex less frequently.[4] That makes sense, because sex is good exercise and its stress-reducing effects can improve sleep and blood pressure. Additionally, sex is a strong motivator for exercise and good diet, which help you look better naked.

- **Lowered prostate cancer risk**—Maybe this is one reason men want so much sex! Multiple studies have shown that men who ejaculate more often enjoy a lower risk of developing prostate cancer than men who ejaculate less frequently.[5] The ejaculation does not have to occur during intercourse, so masturbation offers the same protective effect.

- **Improved sleep**—This may seem obvious if you have ever drifted off after a satisfying session of sex with your partner, but there is evidence that orgasm, whether it comes from sex with a partner or masturbation, leads to better sleep.[6] You will sleep better and peacefully when your mind is fully occupied with sexual fantasies rather than with daytime stress, like dealing with the IRS.

- **Stronger libido**—People engaged in sexual activities will have more sexual thoughts and sexual fantasies, which play an important role in stimulating the libido.

The benefits of sex work both ways. If you are healthier and more vital, you will want and have more sex, but if you have more sex, you are likely to feel better, be healthier, and engage in activities like regular exercise that keep you healthier. That is a win-win!

OUT WITH OUTDATED IDEAS

HOW CAN WE GET TO that point where couples are eager to talk about sex, share their desires and concerns, and openly talk to their doctors about sex with no shame or embarrassment? I think to begin with, we have to let go of some of our outdated ideas about sexuality. They no longer serve us well—on the contrary, they hinder our quality of life.

For example, most religions have long had a problem with sexuality, especially female sexuality. In the Bible, God kicked Adam and Eve out of paradise for seeing each other's nakedness, but it is clear that the book blames Eve because she at the apple, and worse, she pressured Adam to eat it, too. God punished Eve (and all women who come after her) in Genesis 3:16, when he says, "I will greatly multiply thy sorrow and thy conception; in sorrow thou shalt bring forth children; and thy desire shall be to thy husband, and he shall rule over thee."

Shame over sex, and the sense that women's bodies are unclean, is as old as civilization. In ancient Hebrew culture, women had to be apart from their men during their menstrual periods because they were seen as being unclean. The general rule in traditional Judaism is that a man may talk with any woman when she is near her time of the month, but he is not allowed to touch her because she might be near her period. Therefore, while gathering in a place of prayer like a synagogue, the women's section is separated from the men's section, a policy that has created a conflict for people gathering in front of the Wailing Wall in Jerusalem.

Sexual blindness and the idea of women as "unclean" isn't limited by religion, either. In India in early 2019, there were massive protests and riots because two women defied a centuries-old ban on women of menstruation age entering a specific Hindu temple.[7]

The Talmud is more enlightened, offering rules about sex, including acceptable positions, whether the man and woman should meet in day or at night, whether the man is allowed to kiss the woman's sex organs, and so on. The Talmud also states that it is the man's duty to take care of his wife in three aspects: provide her adequate food, give her shelter and clothing, and provide for her sexual needs. The Talmud also specifies that the wife must satisfy her husband sexually before he goes traveling and when he returns.

It's time to do away with the archaic sexual standards and beliefs and accept that loving, generous, open sex between a couple is a blessing. Rejecting that reality ruins health and wrecks marriages, but embracing it enhances health and strengthens the bond between man and woman. It is long past the time to stop assuming that sex is solely natural and happens all by itself. We need to start designing the sexual lives that we as individual couples desire. What does that look like? Well, here is my conception of a physically and mentally healthy sexual life for the average man:

- It is exciting, with some adventurous experimentation with sexual play and a lot of variety. It is a reward that the man must earn from his partner by pleasing her emotionally and physically. He cannot take it without her clear consent. Sex is the motivator to do the right things and tame his urges.

- It is fairly frequent, probably at least once or twice per week, though the amount of sex that makes each couple happy will vary.

- It might feature such elements as open masturbation, role play, or dirty talk, with neither partner feeling shame in this.

- It validates his success and status as a virile provider. This is a relic of our evolutionary past; women were and still are attracted to strong providers and protectors, which explains the frequent age imbalance between men and women. Older men tend to be wealthier and more successful, making them strong providers. Sexual gratification confirms this in the man's mind.

- He is potent in bed, able to satisfy his woman, and this potency translates in other areas, especially his career.

- He feels pride. He is never put in a position where he feels like he has to dominate his woman or beg to get sex. Instead, he has the chance to woo his beloved and feel the thrill of the pursuit.

Over time, we want the man to attach less of his self-worth to his sexual performance and more to his ability to be a mature, compassionate, generous partner in all things. A man who feels this way will be more likely to:

- take care of his body through diet and exercise, staying fit and attractive as he ages, as well as healthy;

- reduce episodes of ED by losing his fear of sexual failure and humiliation;

- take care of his mind through meditation, taking time away from work, and so on. This will reduce the impact of stress and its side effects;

- talk openly about his sexuality with his partner, and teach her what men think and do while learning about women's sexuality;

- see his doctor more often, not neglect or deny symptoms, and be open with his physician about sexual issues;

- maintain a better work-life balance;

- be a more attentive father/grandfather;

- communicate more willingly and honestly with his wife; and

- be understanding and compassionate when his wife doesn't wish to have sex.

In other words, a sexually satisfied man has a chance to be the type of husband most women say they want! But what about the woman? What does a physically and mentally healthy sex life look like for her? As you can imagine from our previous discussions, it does not look the same as that life for a man—and that is as it should be. This is what that life looks like:

- There is a great deal of physical affection—cuddling, hugging, hand holding, and so on. Touch and tenderness mean a great deal for women.

- She feels youthful in spirit, believes in her femininity, and is proud of it.

- She and her husband have plenty of intimate time, which could be spent having sex or just in intimate conversation.

- She feels desired and desirable. This is the counterweight to society's determination that as women age, they become less sexual. All women need to feel desirable, confident, and comfortable with themselves as they grow older. Positive body image should never fade for a woman.

- She is proud of her body and stays sexually active even when her libido is not strong. I have met many women who stay active and interested in sexuality in their seventies and beyond. They are charming, energized, and happy, and they always look self-confident.

- She is in control of the sexual activity in the relationship and enjoys that control but understands her responsibility.

- Because she stays sexually active, she is motivated to take care of her appearance and does not let herself go like women who have let their low libido rule them. She eats right, exercises, manages stress, and dresses attractively.

- She and her husband communicate regularly and candidly about sex.

This woman is strong, confident, and fully aware of the crucial role her sexuality plays in the health and longevity of her marriage. She is comfortable with her own sexuality and places the same importance on her own desires as she does on the desires of her male partner. It's important that the woman's desire always be seen as equally important by both partners. As Vanderbilt University sociologist Heather Hensman Kettrey writes, "Young women's sexual desire and pleasure are viewed as secondary to young men's desires. This can set young women up to accept unwanted advances and participate in undesired sex for the purpose of pleasing a male partner."[8]

Instead, let us strive to have both partners be equal in their love, patience, self-awareness, honesty, compassion, and self-respect.

WHAT A HEALTHY SEX LIFE LOOKS LIKE FOR A COUPLE

THE POWER OF THESE SIMPLE actions is incredible. Communication, trust, and an appreciation for the power and importance of sexuality can overcome even the most difficult relationship challenges. One of my patients, fifty-eight years old, had a mastectomy because of breast cancer. As a result, she would not allow her husband to see her because of her negative body image. She chose not to have cosmetic reconstructive surgery, and she was ashamed of how she looked.

Still, the couple loves each other, and her husband has been incredibly supportive. But the surgery and the negative body image suppressed her libido. Her doctors can't give her hormones because she's had breast cancer, and hormones probably wouldn't help anyway. This is about her self-image—her fear and depression. She does not feel feminine, and that made her libido feel dead.

When I started to talk to her about her self-image, I told her that the best way to recover it was to get back to sexual activity, even if she did not want in the beginning. At first, she would not consider it. People want to find a cause that's outside themselves, something that can be fixed with a shot or a pill. But I kept pressing. "Break the ice," I said. She agreed to try to have sex, and once she started to see her husband coming to her, wanting her, loving her, and reaching orgasm himself, she felt more feminine again. She started to see the light again—her femininity, her value, and her own charm. She began to feel pride in herself again.

With time, she and her husband have gotten back to having sex regularly, and she is like a different person: healthier, happier, more vibrant. That is why sex is like exercise: it has endless benefits that you don't think about when you do it but that you receive anyway. Body image, intimacy, activation of hormones, motivation to be fit—the benefits go on and on and on. Sex is therapeutic.

So, what does a healthy, vibrant, satisfying sex life look like for a healthy couple? Obviously, the definition of that will vary with each couple, but there are some common core elements that I have seen again and again in my practice. Here's an example of a healthy relationship of a couple in their late fifties who have sex once or twice a week:

- They are fit and healthy and often work out and walk together.

- They are usually energetic and participate in a wide range of activities.

- They share similar eating habits and eat a healthy diet, often cooking together.

- They also have interests and hobbies that they pursue independently of one another but talk about with each other.

- They communicate regularly about all sorts of things involving their relationship and home, not just sex.

- They set aside romantic and sexual time for themselves, even going so far as to schedule it on their calendars.

- They play with variety in their sex lives, experimenting with sex in different locations and different positions and trying role play, pornography, oral sex, manual sex, and sex toys. Anything is on the table as long as consent is mutual.

- They discuss fantasies without shame.

- They understand that sometimes, there will be barriers to sex: the man may experience ED from time to time, the woman may have vaginal dryness or low libido, or they may be tired from work. They are patient and understanding when such things happen. Transient failures don't throw them out of balance, force them to quit, or lead to feelings of guilt and shame.

- They approach their sex life with love, humor, and a sense of fun.

- They have a close circle of friends. People enjoy being around them because they are positive and happy.

- They have a strong marriage and family life.

Does that sound like the kind of relationship that you have now? Then you are one of the lucky ones who are doing things right. Does that sound like the kind of relationship you would like to have? Then pursuing a more active, mutually satisfying sex life is one way to achieve it. You see, this is what an adult sex life looks like: rich, fulfilling, honest, communicative, and physically and mentally vibrant.

Want more reasons to pursue better sex? There is research that shows that people who have sex more often earn more money![9] Now, I don't know whether earning more money makes you more attractive, leading to more sex, or if having a lot more sex gives you so much positive energy that you go out and earn more money, but does it matter?

When it is open, passionate, and loving and comes from understanding each other's needs, sex is a pure blessing. More sex and better sex leads to better health, a better marriage, and a better life. Who would not want that?

Chapter Eight

BETTER SEX AS WE AGE? YES!

Some time ago, I met with a new patient, a seventy-eight-year-old woman who had been married for many years to a man around the same age. She acknowledged that her sex drive was strong, but her husband seemed to have lost his, which is unusual even at that age. When I questioned her further, I found out that the underlying problem was her husband's ED. He did not know how to handle it or resolve it, and he kept trying to hide it because of guilt and humiliation. On the surface he pretended that he had no drive so he could avoid situations where he might be embarrassed by his ED. Meanwhile, he was masturbating several times a week in the shower, indicating that his drive was fine.

I eventually convinced his wife to bring him to see me, and we were able to treat his ED, but the point of this story is that sex was very important to this older couple. If you are not yet in your seventies or beyond and you are in a committed relationship when you get to that age, it will be important to you, too. Sexuality remains important to people in the later stages of their lives, and to ignore this reality is to set ourselves up for pain and unhappiness as we age.

Many of my older patients have confirmed that they still have sexual thoughts, fantasies, and urges and that sexual activity is of primary importance for them. Many older men will go far to try to correct their ED, trying all kinds of remedies and even injections before every sexual encounter. Many women will accept these men's actions and even happily participate in anything that keeps their sex lives going.

Because our culture is obsessed with youth and conventional ideas about beauty, we tend to think of sex as something that is off limits to older people. There is this stereotype that while people in their forties and fifties might still be having lots of good sex, by the time men and women get into their seventies, they no longer have an interest in sex. Even if they do, their bodies won't let them try. All the men allegedly have ED, and all the women have low libido. Even thinking about older people—our parents, for example—having sex makes us crinkle up our faces and say, "Yuck."

This is the stereotype of seniors and sex:

- They hold hands, kiss chastely, and pretend they don't care about sex.

- The man is frustrated and secretly masturbates or watches pornography.

- The woman ignores him because her drive is gone and finds other fulfillment in friends and activities.

- They never attempt to have sex.

None of these ideas is true. I have seen thousands of couples past retirement age where the man and woman not only still engaged in sex but craved it, enjoyed it, and savored the love and closeness it brought to their relationship. Sex is never something that older people should surrender; it is one of the joys of living at any age.

There's also this strange belief that older people *shouldn't* care about sex, that it's unseemly and repulsive. That is total nonsense. Sex is not a luxury. Sex is a fundamental human need for both genders and is essential to a healthy relationship and for physical and emotional fuel. It is not just for the young. Many seniors care very much about sex and want to continue having it for as long as they can. I see men in my practice who are in their eighties and want injections into the penis to cure their ED. Their wives are working with them to bring them to orgasm, and they are doing the same for their wives. Sex might not be the same as it was when they were in their forties, but they're trying, and this keeps their sexuality and their relationship strong and vital, while providing the other benefits we mentioned earlier.

Plenty of people in their seventies and beyond are healthy, motivated, and bright, and they want sex. They're not all fading away with Alzheimer's disease. In fact, I've noticed a pattern among my older patients: *the ones who are still having regular, satisfying sex are healthier than the ones who are not.* I think this may have something to do with the ability of sex to improve immune function. Your immune system can crush rocks if you maintain it. It's an incredible ally if you make it work for you. That's why healthy men and women don't go sexually dormant at age forty-two. Women who lose their drive and believe that they are impaired tend to age more quickly; I have seen it. They give up on all the parts of life that used to make them happy.

On the other hand, women who age gracefully are often the ones who match their husbands in their commitment to maintain their sexual energy as they get older. They put on makeup and dress nicely; they exercise and keep fit. Why? They're doing it for sex appeal! They don't want to lose their sex appeal when they age because then they think, "I am worthless because I'm not like the woman I used to be, so why should I take care of myself at all?" Their self-esteem starts to spiral down the drain. For men and women, paying attention to your body and your appearance, and working to maintain sexual activity past middle age and into old age, keeps you feeling good, sexy, and happier.

You know those people past seventy who say, "I don't feel my age?" I will bet that both men and women who say that are still sexually active. I have seen it. In contrast, the ones who tell you, "I feel old; everything is hurting," probably have no sexual activity. Sex both keeps us healthier and tells the world that we're healthier.

"COUPLEPAUSE" AND STAYING SEXUAL TOGETHER

MEDICINE IS BEGINNING TO RECOGNIZE that because sex and aging is an issue that affects *couples*, the man and woman will benefit if they are both treated for sexual dysfunction at the same time. This is a big step. We have long recognized that women in middle age pass through menopause, when their bodies produce less estrogen, they stop menstruating, and they may experience symptoms like reduced libido. But there is also something called the andropause, which refers to men's declining testosterone production—which can lead to ED.

Now, clinicians and sexual medicine specialists are talking about something they call "couplepause." The idea is that couples often experience age-related sexual changes together, so they need to be treated for their dysfunction as a couple. Researchers have found that this enlightened, holistic approach helps older couples achieve more intimacy and greater sexual satisfaction.[1]

Here's my proof: I have a male patient, sixty-eight, who just retired from an engineering company. I have treated him for hypertension and a heart irregularity for several years, and he is medically stable. But over the past four years, he noticed that his energy level had been declining, along with a decrease in his sexual desire and occasional ED. All these symptoms led him to have sex maybe once a month. He lost his drive and his ambition for new projects and felt diminished vigor. He was happy to retire but seemed exhausted and disappointed.

He is devoted to his wife, sixty-two, a retired teacher with mild diabetes, poor sleep, depression, and who had trouble focusing and hot flashes. Neither one had any libido, and at that point there was no excitement in their life. Their children are long gone, and they were planning to have a wonderful postretirement life—traveling, taking cruises, and engaging with sports, dance, and music. Now life is dull, and with the loss of their sex drive, they seem to have lost interest in all those parts of life that used to excite them.

This was a sad story, and I wanted to help them. I realized that going after the wife's symptoms with medication was not the way. Tests showed her to be at the peak of menopause with very low estrogen. After examinations and lab tests, the man was found to have a testosterone deficiency. I suggested that they both start taking hormones, although in itself this would likely be insufficient. To accompany the hormone therapy, I therefore suggested that they also follow a new regimen:

- Exercise daily for at least one hour, preferably together.

- Meet with a dietician for instruction on eating a healthy diet, and lose at least ten pounds in six months.

- Maintain sexual activity at least twice a week.

- Get involved in regular social activities or volunteering.

Three months later, this couple's life has totally changed. The man has regained his full sexual ability and desire. The woman quit seeing endless doctors about her somatic symptoms, reduced her medications, and started to take university classes. After six months, she decided that she could do without her oral estrogen but applied estrogen cream periodically.

The lesson is that while life changes with age, those changes do not need to take away our happiness or fulfillment with all the good things of life including sex. We simply need to pay special attention to our bodies and souls and address our issues with professionals in ways that suit our bodies and our relationships. Had this couple not brought their emotional and sexual problems up for discussion, their lives would have continued to slide. Instead, they were renewed.

The truth is that older people think about sex, want sex, have sex, have sexual thoughts and fantasies, and enjoy the sex they have. Yes, it is true that sexual frequency declines with age, and the longer two people are together and the more familiar they become with each other's bodies and sexual tastes, the more predictable and less exciting sex can become. But there is nothing asexual about the lives of older people.

According to the National Poll on Healthy Aging, roughly 40 percent of men and women ages sixty-five to eighty are sexually active. Predictably, sexual activity decreased with age—only one fourth of those age seventy-six to eighty reported being sexually active, but that is still millions of seniors. Men (51 percent) were more sexually active than women (31 percent), and not surprisingly, people who said that their health was good or excellent were more likely to report satisfying sex lives. Perhaps most telling, 92 percent of people who were sexually active reported that sex is an important part of a romantic relationship.[2]

The last finding is not surprising to me at all. Women and men who have been my patients for years report to me that when they committed to having better sex as they aged, they both enjoyed more individual satisfaction and greater intimacy and closeness in their marriages.

Remember, women and men draw satisfaction from sexuality in different ways. For men, it's mostly about the orgasm but also about the pursuit and the conquest. Even a man in his eighties needs to feel virile and that he can satisfy his wife. For women, sex is more about feeling desired, being close, and satisfying her husband; she doesn't necessarily need an orgasm to find enjoyment in sex. Older couples who understand these differences and account for them in their sex lives are the ones I see who enter their seventies and beyond happy—holding hands, teasing, having great sex, and enjoying their active lives together.

Some of my older patients stay together without sex, living like brother and sister. They support each other through the medical issues that often come up with old age, and that gives them confidence and security. However, the joy of life and the excitement of sex is missed. Medical issues fill most of their daily lives.

When I talk to those couples about resuming sexual activity, I commonly see very positive responses. I have come to the conclusion that inside the minds of all these elderly couples, strong sexual interest still exists. But because of our society's traditions and restrictive discussions about sex, most of these couples will not talk about their desires, and their sexual selves will remain dormant without help. If a physician uses his power to spark that discussion, he can awaken sexuality for the patients and will then deal with healthier patients, fewer repeated symptoms, and fewer prescriptions.

One couple—the man was seventy-six, the woman seventy-two—lived together in a routine, boring life without any sex. Their routine was eating and drinking alcohol. They struggled with various medical problems, including liver disorders from all the drinking, in addition to gaining weight. They never even considered sex as an option.

Change usually happens only when something from outside sparks it and awakens the person; otherwise, programmed routine simply continues. Sometimes, that spark is an unexpected disease that shocks the person into admitting the need for change, but by then, it is often too late. It is much better if the physician takes on the role of truth teller. In helping people acknowledge what is right in front of them that they cannot see, the physician is in a unique role to change lives.

I did that with this couple. I described the harm in their drinking and all the other associated problems it created. I confronted them with the reality of what they were doing to their health. I advised them to quit drinking and instead walk in the neighborhood for one hour daily. They became engaged with hobbies, trips, and social activities. As they started to show motivation, I convinced them to resume their intimate life. Surprisingly, it worked. They lost weight, their livers healed from the alcohol damage, their sleep improved, and their joy from sex returned. Now, they spend their money on travel, not medical care.

THE CHANGES OF AGE DON'T MEAN THE END OF SEX

WHAT I TELL MY PATIENTS is true: if we take care of our bodies and communicate with each other, we can enjoy great sex throughout our entire lives! There is no reason that, with care and attention, a husband and wife can't continue to enjoy this closeness and pleasure.

However, we also must acknowledge that with aging comes inevitable changes to our bodies, and that includes changes that affect desire, arousal, orgasm, and how sex feels. Every age has

REPAIRING SEXUAL DISORDERS POSITIVELY AFFECTS HEALTH AND HAPPINESS

The valuable information that I gain by making sexual inquiries of my patients allows me to help them through an avenue that's completely different from the traditional method of medications. In many cases, this proves much more effective than any medication ever could be.

One example: a fifty-six-year-old man, married for thirty years to a woman now fifty-two. They have one grown son. The man has been my patient for many years, and I have treated him for diabetes, obesity, hypertension, and severe depression. It had been difficult for me to motivate him to watch his diet and exercise, and the lack of excitement in his life did not give him any motivation of his own. He was becoming frustrated and showed signs of giving up. In the past, when I asked him about his sexuality, he acted like it was unimportant but would not give me any more information.

Recently, he came in for a routine follow-up and told me that he just got divorced and moved to an apartment alone and was feeling depressed and helpless. But this time, when I asked him about his sexuality, he opened up and told me a secret he had never told anybody. Thirty years ago, when his wife gave birth to their son, she was attracted to one of the female nurses who attended her and discovered her true sexual orientation. However, because of their child and the social attitude of the time, they both decided to keep the secret from everybody and continue to live with each other as a normal couple—but asexually. Since that time, he had no sexual activity with any woman.

He told me, "I don't even know if I am capable of doing it." He confirmed that he felt completely hopeless about sex and that he masturbated three to four times a week. I jumped on the opportunity to improve his confidence and motivation. I told him that his masturbation indicated that his sexual drive was still healthy and meant that he was good to return to an active sexual life. I suggested that doing so would bring many positive changes to his life.

The man's mood changed immediately. It was as if he had been waiting for someone to give him permission to be a sexual person again. He seemed hopeful and promised that he would act on my advice. Six month later, he came to me again for a follow-up, and he looked different—happy. He had lost twenty-two pounds, his blood pressure was down significantly, and his diabetes was totally controlled. I was able to reduce and eliminate many of his medications.

I asked him about his sex life, and he said, "Doc, I started to go to the gym with a trainer, a beautiful lady, and somehow we became friends, and now she is teaching me how to be a sexual man again."

This case, like many others, showed me that sexuality is a central part of our health, and using it medically, in addition to traditional treatment, can benefit our patients.

its own glory, and we have to adapt to it, work with it, and take advantage of all those stages along with our health. If you want to enjoy sex into old age, the most basic thing you can do is take care of your general health. Every year have a physical with a medical professional who will let you know how your body machine is running. Check your blood pressure, and if it's high, treat it with medication to avoid developing complications. Keep your weight down and exercise to avoid developing type 2 diabetes. Much of this is common sense and entails adopting good lifestyle habits, as well as working with your physician to make sure that all your systems stay in good shape as the years pass.

Of course, your body will change with age. This is unavoidable. The idea is to see these changes not as negatives but simply as your body adapting to the passage of time. There are ways to see sexual change as positive. For example, women who have passed through menopause will say that no longer having menstrual periods or needing to worry about birth control is a load off their minds. They have also gained ample sexual experience and know their own bodies and their partners' bodies better. Being older means there are no children in the house, so you have more freedom to enjoy sex without interruptions and have more time together.

Changes in the body that occur as we age can affect how we desire and experience sex. In men, the changes are things we have already discussed. After age forty, some men will see a gradual drop in their body's production of testosterone, which can affect muscle mass, libido, and of course, the ability to get and maintain an erection. ED can come about as a result of cardiovascular disease and other physiological causes, but it is more often a psychological condition that manifests itself by impairments in performance, as we have seen.

ED does not always mean that a man cannot get an erection. Sometimes, he will take longer to get an erection or his erection may not be as firm as in the past or he may experience premature ejaculation, which can be especially embarrassing if his wife's orgasm is delayed. Some men may take longer to get another erection after achieving orgasm. In all cases, the thing that older men should keep in mind is that no matter the cause, there is almost always a way that ED can be understood and dealt with that will allow the man to keep having sexual relations. That could involve medication, devices like vacuum pumps, or sex through manually stimulating his partner, but the important truth for older men is that ED does not mean the end of sex.

Women experience more age-related sexual changes. In a postmenopausal woman, estrogen levels will drop sharply. As a result, her vagina may shorten and narrow, the vaginal walls can become thinner and stiffer, and her vagina will produce less natural lubrication. This can make sex less enjoyable and even painful, and as you can imagine, the prospect of painful sex can negatively affect the woman's libido. However, this definitely can be addressed as long as you and your partner are open with each other and communicate with your doctor. We cannot treat a condition we don't know exists.

The frequency with which a woman will be able to have sex might have to change to accommodate physical changes, but that is not unexpected with age. Vaginal dryness can be handled using topical hormones (applied to the skin, intravaginally) and commercial lubricants, and sometimes physical positioning makes a difference, allowing the penis to enter at a more comfortable angle.

The key is that even though there are unavoidable physical

changes that come with age, sex can continue—and should continue, since we have seen that it *promotes* good health.

IF YOU ENJOY SEX, CARE FOR YOUR HEALTH

I AM NOT TRYING TO DISCOUNT the effects of aging or the fact that they can make life difficult for some people. The kidneys lose some of their capacity with advanced age even in a healthy person, while lung capacity might decrease as much as 15 percent. We lose 1 percent of our muscle mass every year after age forty, even if we exercise regularly. Growing old, as one man said, is not for sissies.

Time can bring on many physiological changes that can affect sexual functioning:

- **Chronic pain**—If you are suffering from arthritis or general joint pain, you might find sex less pleasurable or difficult. However, even with these difficulties, when a compatible couple determines to continue their sexual activities, they always find a way. Apparently, the power of passion is stronger than any pain. I also notice that these sexually active couples are happier and closer to each other in time of need.

- **Diabetes**—Type 2 diabetes is on the rise in America, driven by a rise in obesity.[3] This disease can damage blood vessels, which in turn impairs arousal in both men and women.

- **Cardiovascular disease**—As we have already talked

about, heart disease narrows blood vessels, blocking the flow of blood to the penis. This is why ED is considered an early warning sign of heart disease or diabetes, especially in young men.

- **Obesity**—Research says obesity appears to interfere with sex for older women but not older men.[4]

- **Cancer and cancer treatment**—Cancer itself can cause symptoms that make sex undesirable, and the stress of a cancer diagnosis can diminish desire. Also, treatments such as chemotherapy can leave a person feeling too ill to care about sex.

- **Stress incontinence**—With age, some women become more likely to lose bladder control under certain conditions, and this can make sex embarrassing, which impairs libido.

- **Neurological conditions**—Conditions ranging from multiple sclerosis to stroke to spinal cord injury can upset the delicate coordination of brain, hormones, and muscles that lead to desire and arousal.[5]

- **Dementia**—One in seven Americans over age seventy has dementia[6], and this can change the sexual feelings and thoughts of the person with dementia, potentially interfering with desire and performance. I have seen men with dementia exhibit inappropriate sexual talk and expressions that are very unpleasant to witness. So write in your will, "Please don't believe what I say when I have dementia."

How well we take care of our bodies makes all the difference between reaching age eighty with health and vitality and an enjoyable sex life and reaching that same age with crippling illness and life devoid of sex. Research has shown that men and women who engage in good lifestyle choices—exercising, maintaining a healthy weight, not smoking, and eating a diet rich in healthful foods—had a life expectancy twelve to fourteen years longer than people who didn't adopt any of the low-risk lifestyle factors.[7] In other words, living long and living well is less about our genes and more about our choices, and that includes sex.

I have seen many couples in their seventies with beautiful marriages and an enjoyable sexual life who took care of their health and took responsibility for it by making good choices. They exercise. They look after their blood pressure and cholesterol. They watch what they eat. They get enough sleep. They keep their minds busy, even in retirement. This keeps their energy high, and that's important because your libido depends a great deal on your happiness, on your satisfaction in life in general, and on your mood. So set a lifetime of good sex as a goal and then keep working toward it. Keep finding ways to keep desire burning.

The fact is that not all age-related physical changes are inevitable for all people, and some can be delayed or avoided with good lifestyle choices. There are also positive changes that come with age that can improve sex, including greater closeness and intimacy, better knowledge of what you and your partner like in bed, more time for sex, and greater confidence. I have seen older patients take great delight in defying the expectations of younger people (including their children) by continuing to have robust sex lives. That is a fine goal to have!

Here is another couple that demonstrates this point. Both were happily married for more than forty years, and they were mutually supportive and sexually very active. The man developed terminal cancer and was placed on chemotherapy. They continued supporting and loving each other to the end. After her husband died, it took the woman a year to mourn, but after that, she returned to life and regained her confidence. She went on dates with older men. She took care of her appearance, dressed attractively, and assertively looked for a sexually active man who would love her and treat her tenderly. That intention, belief, and strength came because of her previous experience, knowing that sex was important to her whole life. I admire this woman!

Good Sex Means Different Things to Different People

There is no gold standard for "right" when it comes to sex after age fifty. It is whatever works for you and your partner. Experts agree that sex into old age can be just as hot and satisfying as sex when you are younger, but that looks different for everyone. For men, who maintain their libido well into old age, sex once a month or more plus masturbation might work just fine. Who cares, as long as you are happy and satisfied? There is no right amount or right kind of sexual satisfaction.

For women, I like the words of author Iris Krasnow, who said in an interview with SeniorPlanet.com, "Sexuality matters to us until the day we die. How we manifest that is different for every woman. There is no gold standard. There is no perfect sex life. What matters the most is how you feel about your sexuality, your level of desire and your libido. You want to communicate your sexual expectations, desires, and performance levels to your partner and for your partner to be on the same page. Problems arise when you don't match. There are women who are postmenopausal, have lost their libido and don't want to be on hormones or use the 'vaginator' that stretches female sex organs. There were a few women I interviewed who were in intimate relationships with men whose libido matched theirs. They had zero interest in sex and were happy just hiking in the woods."[8]

In other words, whatever makes you and your partner happy is "right."

ELDER SEX HAS ITS BENEFITS TOO

THE OTHER GOOD NEWS IS that even when you're in your seventies or beyond, having sex is beneficial to your body! We have already touched on some of the proven health benefits of staying busy sexually, but there are some that are particularly meaningful to people beyond retirement age.

First of all, sex is great exercise that burns fat and aids the cardiovascular system. Some cardiologists say that a session of intercourse is like climbing several flights of stairs, and I agree. Also, for women, sex is like physical therapy for incontinence because it works the muscles and tendons of the pelvic floor, which can weaken with age and lead to urinary problems. For both partners, more frequent sex—including kissing, cuddling, and fondling—is associated with greater enjoyment of life. Women seem to care more about intimacy, while men care more about intercourse, but for both genders, sex leads to greater happiness.[9]

Sex also stimulates the release of human growth hormone in both men and women, and this can help keep skin elastic, reduce wrinkles, firm muscles, and improve the look of hair, leading to more confidence, better body image, and more desire for sex. Having sex also may prevent cancer of the prostate, perhaps by stimulating its function. In other words, the more you use the parts of your body that were designed for sex, the readier for sex you will be.

The reality is that we can continue having great sex into old age, but we have to be realistic about our expectations. I have seen many couples in my office who had wonderful sex lives into old age, and all of them had one thing in common: they did not make the mistake of assuming that sex at seventy-five would be the same as sex at forty. They adapted, communicated, and made adjustments. They rolled with the punches.

For instance, with age, most women have delayed orgasms. It takes them longer to reach climax, and the man needs to maintain his erection for a longer period of time so she can reach her orgasm. However, as we know, a high percentage of women do not reach orgasm from intercourse alone, so the man should not obsess about bringing his lady to climax this way. As the man grows older, he probably will not be able to maintain his erection for as long as he did when he was young, so he should learn about the female physiology and become comfortable with stimulating his wife in other ways. As always, the key is communicating with each other, talking to your physician, and finding encouragement in the truth that there is always hope.

A PRESCRIPTION FOR ENJOYING SEX INTO YOUR EIGHTIES . . . AND BEYOND

ONE OF THE PARTS OF my practice that brings me the greatest pleasure is helping a couple get past sexual problems and then watching them walk together into old age still loving one another, being affectionate, and enjoying the benefits of a fulfilling sexual life. Not all couples are able to do this, but the ones who are open and honest with each other and who take care of their bodies have a much greater chance of being blessed. I believe that most couples at advanced ages can continue with sexual activity if they wish, but they will need to communicate and be consistent.

The other thing that such couples have in common is that many of them have had to work to rekindle their sexual desire after it's disappeared. Remember, for women especially, the key to restoring libido is often having sex even when the desire is not present, and while that is true for women in their forties and fifties, it is even more true for women in their sixties and seventies. Meanwhile, ED becomes more common for men as the years pass. As we age, more conditions pile up that can affect both women's and men's sexuality, so restarting sex in the later years is not as easy. But it is *not* impossible! When you speak to each other with love, when you make time for caresses and stimulation, when you do whatever you must to reach orgasm, the effects will be overwhelmingly positive.

In the seventies or eighties, this will take time. It will take patience. It could take the help of pills, injections, lotions, or devices, and if you have never used them before, you might be uncomfortable. But it is a faulty expectation that is making you uncomfortable—the expectation that sex in old age should be the same as sex in your youth. *It won't be.* Accept that now and open yourself to trying new things to keep those fires roaring. They really do work, as long as you and your partner are open minded and love each other enough to try.

What does a great sex life in old age look like for a man? Here are some thoughts:

- feeling younger than his actual age, something that is closely associated with higher self-esteem and happiness

- enjoying sex more, even if it is not as frequent

- not feeling the pressure to bring his female partner to orgasm through intercourse each time because he understands her physiology and is comfortable with using other means to make her climax when achievable

- being comfortable with the use of sex toys, lubricants, and other sexual aids that in the past might have threatened his manhood

- being comfortable with experimentation

- being adept at compensating and adjusting for health-related challenges to sex

- keeping a healthy libido

- being motivated to exercise and keep his body fit and strong

- feeling a strong sense of self-confidence and masculinity

- making time for sex

Overall, men who enjoy healthy sex lives into their later years feel powerful and virile, something that many older men do not. They are much happier in their relationships in part because they feel like they are defying the stereotype that "old people don't have sex." They feel rebellious, audacious, and powerful. They enjoy life and enjoy taking care of their wives.

What about women? What does a satisfying, rich sexual life in their seventies and eighties look like for them? As we have said many times, the two machines are different, so their markers of happiness and satisfaction are somewhat different . . . but not all of them are. Here is what I have seen among women:

- They also feel younger than their calendar age, which is associated with higher self-esteem and happiness.

- They also enjoy sex more, even when it is not as frequent as in the past.

- They deeply enjoy the physical closeness, feelings of femininity and of being special, and sense that they are still attractive that come with sex in their later years. By this time, couples know each other very well and have adapted to each other's needs, so the emotional side of their sex is deep and rich.

- They usually enjoy improved libido, along with ambition and motivation.

- They are more likely to remain sexually active because they engage in positive behavior like eating a good diet, exercising, dressing attractively, and engaging socially with their husbands. They will spend time, money, and energy to take care of themselves.

- They will continue to reach orgasm, though probably not during every sexual encounter.

- They are, like their husbands, comfortable with the use of sexual aids.

- They enjoy the idea that they are sexier and more sexually adventurous than their peers.

Women who enjoy satisfying sex in old age reject the notion that getting older automatically means the loss of sexual desire and with it the loss of sexual closeness and feeling like a woman. They reject the notion that life with their partner has to be dull, mechanical, and routine. Instead, they fight past low libido and engage in sex as a way to experience pleasure and stimulate their sexual bodies. They feel better, look better, and have closer, more loving marriages.

What might a good sex life look like for an older couple? I will share with you the story of the parents of a gentleman I know. They are not my patients, but they are a wonderful example of how, with love and understanding, sex remains not only possible but good into our later years.

This gentleman told me that his parents, who were open with him about intimacy and both in their seventies and married for more than fifty years, continue to enjoy a terrific sex life despite many health challenges. His father, who is overweight, has experienced a series of recurring and very dangerous leg infections over the past few years, and that has left his mobility very limited. His mother spends many hours each day caring for her husband, who cannot walk well, and dressing the recurrent wounds on his legs. So, despite being healthy, she is exhausted. They spend several days each month at hospitals getting the husband's legs attended to—and if an infection flares up, time in the emergency room. This has made their lives very stressful.

However, despite all this, they have a fulfilling, loving sex life. First of all, they have chosen to make sex a priority. They talk about it, tease about it, and make time for it. The husband's mobility is poor, so they have had to change the way they have sex from the way they had it for years when he was healthy. They have found ways to satisfy each other, bring each other to orgasm, and enjoy the physical and emotional satisfaction that comes with sexuality, all in spite of challenges that might make other couples give up completely. Because of this, even with the challenges they face, they remain mentally sharp, happy, and devoted to each other.

WHAT GREAT SEX INTO OLD AGE REQUIRES

I LOVE TO HEAR STORIES like that one because they let me know that it is not only my patients who are breaking the stereotypes of age and sex. Millions of people around the country are savoring great sex many years after retirement age. You can do the same thing! However, there are a few things you must do to gain admission to this exclusive club:

- Make sex a priority in your lives. Do not take it for granted or assume it will "take care of itself." Have a plan and communicate with each other.

- Adopt habits now that will delay the onset of chronic disease and keep you healthy. Don't smoke. Exercise at least five hours a week. Eat a diet rich in healthy fruit, vegetables, nuts, seeds, and lean proteins. Take supplements that have been found to have value, like antioxidants and fiber. Manage your job stress. Get enough sleep.

- Establish an open relationship with a personal physician who is happy to talk with you about your sex life, and keep that conversation going.

- Have sex as much as possible. Talk about it. Schedule

it. Learn about your body and your partner's body and become better at sex.

- Address any problems proactively. Talk about ED or low libido. See your doctor for suggestions and to rule out causes. Talk to a sex therapist. Don't let things go; address them.

The recurring message of this book is that there is hope for virtually anyone experiencing problems with sex, and that applies here as well. There is tremendous hope for couples who want to enjoy vibrant, fun, stimulating sex into their seventies and beyond. As with so many other aspects of health and well-being, the outcome is entirely in your control.

Chapter Nine

TIME TO
BREAK
THE TABOO

I think by now we have established beyond a doubt that sex is beneficial for overall health, the health of the marriage, and the mental health of men and women. It is not a luxury. It is not dirty or sinful. Sex is a basic need, a vital part of who we are, a gift from nature to humans. So why can we still not talk about sex and sexuality like adults?

Sex education in the United States is a constant topic of conflict and argument. Enlighted parents believe, correctly, that their children should know everything about their sexuality so they can make better decisions and avoid negative outcomes like sexually transmitted infections (STIs) and unwanted pregnancy, not to mention sexual violence. Other parents mis-

takenly think that sex is bad and dangerous and that giving information to their kids just makes them promiscuous and encourages
premature sex. They feel that their children are better off knowing
as little as possible about sex. As a result, we have a patchwork
of state laws and even different policies within different schools,
and millions of young people come into adulthood knowing little
or nothing about this vital part of being human.

We evolve into who we are as adults from our experiences in
childhood and beyond. So we have to educate ourselves about sex
from a young age. Be open about it with each other. Only through
open discussion and teaching can we learn how sex can make us
happy and learn to handle its power. But in school right now, if
the school offers sex education at all, they might talk about birth
control, the menstrual cycle, how pregnancy occurs, and STIs.
Today, some schools might use a banana to show boys how to put
a condom on, but that never happened when I was growing up.

While the schools are important, it is the parents who really
need to take responsibility. Parents have more authority over their
children than any teacher ever will. If you have children, they trust
you and will listen to you. They will learn from watching you. The
more comfortably and openly you discuss sex with your partner,
the more your children will think, "Wow, sex isn't an issue I should
be afraid to bring up." But that is not what happens in many homes.
Instead, parents say, "We don't want the schools teaching our children about sex. That's something that we should be doing at home."
But then they don't do it at home. So the children learn nothing.

Whatever a child is told, learning will be affected by the environment. I have noticed when dealing with patients suffering from
chronic severe anxiety associated with panic disorders, there is
always a childhood background to it. They never understand it and

can't explain it, but when I ask them about their parents, they will usually tell me that one of them was an anxious, nervous person. That shows how the environment at home transmits a feeling to the child, even without talk. When the child grows up in a home where the parents love each other, are compassionate, sexually active, and content, that child will be more likely to grow up with a healthy attitude about sex.

Demonstrate love for children by being physically close to each other, touching each other affectionately, and touching your child in the same way. On the other hand, if you demonstrate fear, shame, and secrecy about sex, the child will absorb that lesson and treat sex with the same taboo that afflicts so many people in our society.

The reluctance that people today have for talking openly about sexuality reflects their parents' unease at talking about it. Some of this comes from their religious tradition because many religions teach people that sex is bad, evil, sinful, and so on. If you learn that as a child, you might assume that sex is something that you should never talk about, under any circumstances. You might forbid your children from mentioning it. You might put them in a school that teaches abstinence, an approach that has been proven not to work.[1] In any case, you don't talk about sex with your partner or your children, and the result is a family that is sexually dysfunctional.

Instead, let me tell you what I would like to see in families. The father will sit with his daughters and tell them about how his sexual systems work. The mother will sit with her sons and openly tell them about her sexuality. Then, the father and the mother would sit with the kids together, openly share experiences, and answer questions. Nothing would be off the table. Can you imagine how much misinformation would be prevented, and how much closer the family would become by talking with so much candor and respect?

Young people today certainly don't think about their parents having sex. They either think about the idea as dirty or don't think about it at all. That just teaches them that sex is shameful and that sex should not be a part of getting older. It is better if we give young people a positive example and a model of good sex through the affection, unity, and passion of their parents. In other words, *you are the best lesson.* When a child doesn't see the positive aspects of their parents' sexuality, they don't get a healthy model for their own lives; this will ultimately turn out to be an educational failure that leaves important gaps in the child's self-development and confidence in their own sexuality. It is essential that children get guidance from their parents to help them navigate future relationships.

We must break the taboo. Because when something has mystery around it, when it is forbidden, what is the first thing that young people want to do? They want to break the taboo, and without proper preparation and experience, they will make the mistakes their parents tried to prevent by making sex a taboo in the first place: unwanted pregnancy, STIs, and more. But when you demystify sex, the taboo is gone. Now they know what gives them those funny feelings down there and up here, and they know the risks because they were adequately prepared. They have received good guidance from their parents and are less likely to feel the need to rebel.

I know a gentleman whose father taught him to drink when he was sixteen years old. The father would pour beer for his son at home, drink with him, and teach him about the effects of the alcohol, what it felt like to become a little drunk, and so on. They would drink whiskey and do the same thing. The son was safe because he was at home, and not only was he learning about alcohol, but the mystery and the taboo were being taken away. The father, who was very wise, knew that by doing this, he was reducing the chance that his son would drink out of rebellion and possibly get himself hurt or killed. He made the experience positive.

I would like to see us do the same with sex. Take away the mystery and the forbidden nature of it. Let our children know that sex is for reproduction as well as for pleasure and for enjoyment. Talk about how it is a positive power in our lives, but also talk about its negative aspects. Treat it with respect. If you have an issue, bring it to your partner and your physician. Break the secrecy. When I started asking my patients about their sex lives, it was like a dam breaking; they were hungry to talk and be heard. What if you and your spouse were the ones saying, "Hey, Doc, let's talk about my sex life for a while."

That would end the secrecy and the shame. It would help physicians learn and take better care of their patients. It would do away with so many of the myths and misconceptions that hurt us in our lives and marriages. We would learn that low libido in women is common and normal, but that women can have very satisfying sex and even enjoy orgasm without the initial desire. We would learn that low female libido does not have to mean the end of sex in the marriage. We would learn that ED is common in men and not something that should spark shame or humiliation. It is not a disease and may be just a transient symptom. Men would quickly discover that there are many ways to deal with ED.

Seventy percent of my male patients with ED, when I help them find their confidence, stop experiencing ED. The other 30 percent, those who have physiological causes, get help working around the causes. If they have diabetes, we control their diabetes. If they need Viagra, I give them Viagra to break the fear and start the momentum. If they have a testosterone deficiency, they will get testosterone. For the ones with nerve damage, we find another way for them to enjoy sex. When the conversation is open and mature, anything is possible.

I have a female patient, fifty years old, happily married to a great husband and father. I wondered why she was so happy. When I asked her about sex, she was open and willing to answer any question related to her intimate life. She said that she and her husband have sex three times a week or more, and she stressed to me that she never rejects his sexual advances. "I know how much men need sex," she said to me, "and besides, I enjoy it as well, and it ends up working for both of us." She told me that they have a nineteen-year-old daughter, and she was already sharing her sexual views with her daughter.

My conversation with this lady was enlightening, and I have since shared it with other female patients. But this woman's attitude is not common. Most of the women I see don't understand male sexuality and are frequently confused about how to respond to their man's sexual advances. Some see it as a threat, an insult, or a humiliation, depending on their background and self-confidence. I thought this lady's approach was the healthiest I had seen in a long time. By doing what was good for her husband, she was also doing what was good for herself!

Talking openly about sexuality will change our lives. So let's look at how we can do that.

WE HAVE TO CHANGE THE CULTURE

WHEN MY PATIENTS TELL ME that they are having sexual problems that are threatening their marriage and their happiness, the most common reason for the problems is that they are not communicating about sex. In fact, most of these couples have never communicated with each other about sex, apart from the basics like, "Are you in the mood, honey?" I would say that a majority of my patients never talk with their partners about each other's desires, preferences, and concerns.

That doesn't make any sense. Would you go to see a barber or hair stylist who didn't ask you what you wanted your hair to look like and just began cutting? Of course not. So why would anyone spend decades with another person, sharing the most intimate life imaginable, and not speak explicitly about what they like and dislike in bed, what positions cause them discomfort, what brings them to orgasm, what they have always wanted to try and so on?

The American reluctance to talk about sex is strange to people like me, who grew up in other cultures, or to the Europeans, who are more frank and open about sex. I suspect it comes from the Puritanical roots of this country, as well as the association of sex with being unclean and immoral. Everything was about getting into heaven, and the only way to do that was through hard work and self-denial.

As a result, America has grown up with a two-sided sexual culture—two faces of sexuality, if you want to look at it that way. On one hand, we don't talk about sex, certainly not in the confines of the romantic relationship or marriage. Couples are supposed to know by instinct what the other person likes in bed, and if there is something wrong such as ED or a low libido, each partner is supposed to know that too. However, we don't talk about those problems; they are supposed to solve themselves. None of it makes any sense because the sexual problems between a man and woman rarely solve themselves. Instead, they fester into anger, resentment, fear. They destroy relationships. Silence, not infidelity, kills marriages.

The other face of American sexual culture is our obsession with impersonal, exploitative sex. Unable to talk about sex with our loved ones, we consume it through internet pornography; popular culture in the form of magazines, TV shows, and movies; and dating services like Tinder that make it easy for people to "hook up" for casual sex with no intimacy.

All this turns sex into a transaction instead of the most intimate, meaningful form of connection two people can share. I think the reason is that because of things like the internet, television, and phones, we have become afraid of each other. People no longer talk to their neighbors; they watch Netflix. They no longer talk with their children because everyone is on a smart phone. We get food delivered because we don't want to go to restaurants. We don't like to interact with each other, and no interaction is more intense than sex. We are afraid of the vulnerability and honesty of having and talking about sex, so we avoid both.

The key to change is giving us safe opportunities to talk about sex in the open—having adult conversations about sex that treat sex as a biological need, an important component of human wellness, and nothing to be ashamed of.

WHAT WE SHOULD BE TALKING ABOUT

DR. BENJAMIN SPOCK, WHO WROTE the bestselling book *Dr. Spock's Baby and Child Care*, got this issue right when he said, "Sex education, including its spiritual aspects, should be part of a broad health and moral education from kindergarten through grade twelve, ideally carried out harmoniously by parents and teachers."

However, getting to that point will take some work. This is what the authors of a study published in the *Journal of Adolescent Health* wrote about the state of sex education in this country:

> *The Centers for Disease Control and Prevention's 2014 School Health Policies and Practices Study found that high school courses require, on average, 6.2 total hours of instruction on human sexuality, with 4 hours or less on HIV, other sexually transmitted infections (STIs), and pregnancy prevention. Moreover, 69% of high schools notify parents/guardians before students receive such instruction; 87% allow parents/guardians to exclude their children from it. Without coordinated plans for implementation, credible guidelines, standards, or curricula, appropriate resources, supportive environments, teacher training, and accountability, it is no wonder that state practices are so disparate.[2]*

We are treating sex education as optional when it is not. Parents often do this out of fear, but Dr. Spock also debunked parental fears that sex education would lead to their children having more sex when he said, "Does sex education encourage sex? Many parents are afraid that talking about sex with their teenagers will be taken as permission for the teen to have sex. Nothing could be further from the truth. If anything, the more children learn about sexuality from talking with their parents and teachers and reading accurate books, the less they feel compelled to find out for themselves."

That is true. Where do young people get their answers about sex when their parents don't teach them? They ask their peers (who probably don't know much more than they do), search the Internet, and read pornographic magazines. They also learn through experimentation, and that can lead to unfortunate consequences. In fact, not educating young people about sex—and not creating an environment in the home and at school where they are encouraged to ask questions—can lead to some ridiculous myths, such as the following:

- Squeezing lemon juice on a person's genitals can tell you if they have an STD.

- If you have sex in a swimming pool, you can't get pregnant.

- Masturbation causes blindness and brain damage.

- Birth control pills cause cancer.

Those are just some of the silly things people believe about sex, but they are not so silly if you have never been told otherwise. Talk about sex in our culture needs to be frank, true, open, encouraged, comprehensive, and mature. This is not a subject for snickering and making jokes; this is a subject that affects lives, marriages, and families. These are the issues that should be on the table for parents, educators, therapists, and physicians—important issues that will affect your kids' futures and happiness:

- **Pregnancy**—Obviously, this is the greatest risk from sex. While it is not a likely outcome for people over fifty years of age, unwanted pregnancy is certainly a risk for younger people, and it can ruin the lives of young women who have babies before they are ready. Girls who give birth as adolescents are more likely to have serious health problems, not complete high school, end up in poverty, and have dangerous clandestine abortions than women who have wanted pregnancies when they are older.[3] And obviously, a young girl becoming pregnant often leads to a baby who ends up in the foster care system.

  Giving young men and women complete information about how pregnancy happens and how to prevent it, as well as debunking myths, will do a great deal to prevent misery for women and men who should have their whole lives ahead of them.

- **Fertility**—According to the US Department of Health and Human Services, 12 to 13 percent of couples in the United States have some trouble conceiving a child.[4] However, many couples do not understand the causes of male and female infertility. It's not because you rode your bike too much or spent too much time in the hot tub. Couples who have the facts can work with great doctors to increase their chances of conception, but first, we have to give them the facts, including sound information on sexual practices that give them the best chance of conceiving.

- **Sex education**—Comprehensive sex education reduces the incidence of unintended pregnancy and STIs.[5] By contrast, there is no evidence that so-called AOUM (Abstinence Only Until Marriage), which exists only to satisfy conservative religious groups, does anything to reduce the rates of pregnancy or disease.

In fact, it's just the opposite: a study that looked at pregnancy rates for women ages fifteen to nineteen between 1998 and 2016 found that not only is abstinence-only education ineffective in decreasing teenage pregnancies, but teen pregnancies in conservative states that focused on AOUM actually *increased*.[6] I believe this is because when we teach abstinence we reinforce the taboo of sex, which makes teens only want to investigate more, often with unfortunate outcomes.

- **Birth control**—Yes, birth control prevents pregnancy, helps couples plan their families, and gives women greater control over their bodies. However, those are not its only benefits. Research shows that widely available birth control has led to higher wages for women, allowed more women to apply to and enter college and earn advanced degrees, and led to healthier children.[7] People need to be educated on the various types of birth control: how effective they are, their possible risks and side effects, their safety, and how to use them properly. We should be teaching children and adults about:

  - » oral contraceptives—how to get them, what they do and don't do, potential side effects
  - » condoms—different types, why they work, how to use them properly

- » IUDs—the benefits of this form of contraception, which in some cases can be hormone-free
- » diaphragm—how to use it, when to remove it, how to use it with spermicide
- » hormone patches, shots, and implants—introduce hormones into a woman's body that prevent the sperm from reaching the egg to fertilize it or prevent ovulation. Each offers protection for a different length of time, so it's important for each woman to understand how long she wants to prevent conception.
- » vasectomy—a simple outpatient surgical procedure that severs the vas deferens, which transports sperm to mix with seminal fluid that comes out when a man ejaculates. A vasectomy effectively makes a man permanently infertile but does not cause ED.

- **Sexually transmitted infections**—People of all ages get them, and people over forty-five have shown the highest rates of increase in STIs in recent years, presumably because they think they don't need to take precautions.[8] This clearly points to the need for educating people of all ages on what the most common STIs are, how they are transmitted, the most high-risk forms of sex, ways of preventing infection, and how these diseases can be treated. The fact that gonorrhea and other infections have become more common recently means we are clearly not doing enough.

- **Sexual violence and harassment**—We live in the #MeToo era, when more and more people are becoming aware of sexual behavior that oversteps safe boundaries and makes people—primarily women—feel unsafe or offended. Our conversation and education should address what is acceptable and unacceptable behavior for men and women and address the fact that making sex taboo and not talking about it—not acknowledging the need for it, especially in men—has led to a culture of secrecy, shame, rage, and violence.

Vasectomy Myths

Men in general are more squeamish about seeing the doctor than women, and they are certainly more reluctant to talk about anything that suggests a lack of sexual potency. That is why so many men seem to fear the idea of having a vasectomy. But this is completely unnecessary! Vasectomy is a safe outpatient procedure that usually takes a urologist less than one hour to perform. Men go home right away, rest for a day or two, submit a sample of semen to ensure that the procedure has worked, and that's it.

In India, this procedure is performed with a sort of assembly line as a way to control population growth. Men stand in line, prepared for the procedure, and the doctor moves from one to the next to perform the surgery.

Performed properly, a vasectomy will not interfere with your ability to get an erection, will not reduce your testosterone level, and should not interfere with your sexual performance or enjoyment of sex in any way. In fact, some men report that they enjoy sex more because they and their wives no longer need to worry about birth control! If you are a man and you and your wife do not want more children, consider having a vasectomy. It is a wonderful gift that you can give your precious wife.

HOW DO WE DO THIS?

OF COURSE, THERE IS A long way to go in getting from where we are today to talking openly, and even enthusiastically, with our partners, teachers, and children about sex. Sex remains a subject for snickers in the hallways and hidden websites. I see nearly every day in my medical practice how the inability of mature adults to talk freely about sex with each other—even though they may have shared a bed for forty years—cripples their relationships and families. Things need to change, and that change needs to begin now.

First of all, I would like to see improved school sexual education programs. Defund abstinence programs. Get involved with organizations like Advocates for Youth, which among other things, promote comprehensive sex education for children. Be aware of groups like StopCSE.org, which insist that comprehensive sex education is harmful to the innocence of our children (whatever that means; this is similar to the movement against vaccination) and tries to prevent schools from setting up honest, science-based sex education curricula. Talk to members of your school board and state legislature and your congressional representatives about expanding the availability of quality sex education in the schools, starting in middle school.

If you attend a church that stigmatizes sexuality and shames people who are sexually active, make your voice heard. Many of our most restrictive, damaging attitudes about sex come from religious teachings, but through compassionate dialogue within your religious community, maybe you can reach confidence in your own sexuality and attitude toward sex. And if you cannot get your church to tone down its anti-sex rhetoric, consider going to another church.

Show your support for political candidates and legislation that promise to make things like contraception and sex education more widely available. Talk willingly with your physician about sexual issues—performance problems, libido, orgasm, birth control, fertility, anything. Do not be afraid to ask the hard questions, and if your doctor is not comfortable answering them, find a new doctor.

Finally, make your home a safe place for talk about sex, whether that is between you and your partner, among your children, or between you and your kids. Let everyone know your house is a "taboo-free zone" where any question is fair game: oral sex, anal sex, masturbation, sex toys, sex myths, losing one's virginity, pregnancy, how the body works, menstruation, and so on. Have books, websites, or videos on hand to answer questions that you can't answer. Make it clear that as far as you are concerned, there is no topic that is off limits and no question that will not be treated with respect.

Can you imagine how much less misinformation about sex there would be—not just among teens but among middle-aged adults—if we spoke about sex that freely and unselfconsciously? If information was available on demand and no fifteen-year-old boy had to feel embarrassed about asking his dad, "Is it okay for me to masturbate?" Educating ourselves about sex, doing away with the taboos, and giving us and our children what we all need to make better sexual choices will give everyone the best chance at a brighter, healthier, happier future.

Chapter Ten

THE
BASHFUL
PHYSICIAN

We have come nearly to the end of the road, but there is one more part of this picture of healthy sex and happier relationships that we still need to address. That is the role of the physician. I have been practicing medicine for more than forty-five years, and as I have said, I have learned far more from my patients than I ever learned from my classes or my textbooks in medical school. Medical school can teach a young man or woman how the lymphatic system functions and how beta-amyloid plaques form in the brain to cause Alzheimer's, but that is teaching someone little more than biology and organic chemistry, like teaching a mechanic how a car's engine functions.

However, if we total the entire knowledge contained in medicine, it will not come to more than about 5 percent of what really happens within our bodies. So, my dear fellow physicians, be careful not to be carried away by the illusion that you know everything and can do everything. We need to be humble, acknowledge the fact that we know very little about the marvelous human body, and try to use what we do know to do good for our patients while being open to learning more.

Additionally, acknowledging the power of nature in the human body and learning to use it for the patient's benefit in addition to what we know will give us a wider range of capabilities to become better physicians than simply relying on diagnostic tests. This is about teaching medical students to be healers who observe, sense, feel, listen, and question the real human beings who come into their offices and who respect their incredible bodies.

If we want more men and women to speak openly about their sexual dysfunction and to seek the help that can make them happier and save families, we need physicians to stop being embarrassed to talk about sex. We need physicians to start talking with their patients about their sex lives. There are two main reasons that they don't do this. First, they are uncomfortable with the topic. Perhaps they are afraid of being seen as inappropriate, or perhaps they were raised in a home where sex was not talked about and was a taboo topic. Consequently, they discard the subject altogether and dive into the usual review of systems.

The second reason is that most physicians aren't trained in sexuality. Think about the position that a young, new physician is in. He or she has just spent four years as an undergraduate, four years in medical school, passed multiple licensing exams, spent three years in a residency, and passed his or her board certification.

By the time he or she does all this and is finally ready to practice with real patients, he or she might be thirty years old. Over the past twelve years, he or she has worked basically nonstop, with little time for dating or sex, much less a real relationship. Suddenly, a patient walks into his or her office and expects him or her to be an expert on marital stresses and sexuality? It's impossible.

The more we spend time learning about something, the more comfortable we are with it, and that is most certainly true of doctors-in-training when it comes to sexuality. If we as physicians are going to lead this revolution of sexual openness and healthy thinking about sex, we need to learn about what sex means to us and to the people we want to help. That change begins in the country's medical schools.

Medical educators must acknowledge that human sexuality is just as important and vital as the endocrine or cardiovascular systems. Schools must teach the sexual system's vital connection with all other systems and integrate it with overall evaluation of the patient's other medical disorders.

FROM CLINICAL TO HUMAN

THE TYPICAL MEDICAL SCHOOL CURRICULUM does not approach medicine from a holistic point of view, and in the beginning, that is understandable. The goal early on is to teach the young student about the basic physiological and biochemical systems and processes that govern the human body as we know it: the neurobiology of the brain, the conversion of polypeptides into amino acids and then back into proteins, and so much more.

The human body is unbelievably complex, and there is so much to learn that it isn't surprising that schools and students are consumed with simply getting all this raw data across.

But after that learning is done, what then? Well, in most cases medical schools are content to treat students as gifted auto mechanics, and that includes the way that they teach them about sexuality. Most medical schools treat sex as coldly as they do kidney disease. They do not teach students anything about the importance of talking to the patient or developing intimacy and trust. They certainly don't teach anything about how stress can affect sexual desire or performance or how the terrible stress and depression that comes with sexual dysfunction affects a patient's mental, behavioral, and physiological health. Instead, lessons focus primarily on:

- how the reproductive system works and what can impair it;

- how and why ED happens, and what it may indicate for the health of the patient;

- how vaginal dryness, menopause, and female loss of libido happen; and

- sexually transmitted diseases.

That's it. The sexual curriculum is all about disease: ED related to atherosclerosis, low libido related to menopause or hypothyroid, and the like. There is no talk about how sex affects overall health or mental health, how it affects motivation, behavior, habits, relationships, sleep, or lifestyle choices. There is no talk about how sexual dysfunction can increase the risk of depression and anxiety. And there is no talk about the ways having frequent sex makes men and women say they enjoy life more and are happier.

Medical school students (and later on, physicians) don't focus on their patients being happy; they only care about making the right diagnosis. People become pathologies, dead tissue under the microscope. While it's important to fix broken bone and torn muscle, what about fixing a broken family and traumatized kids? Sorry, that is too messy and imprecise, so schools and doctors don't deal with it.

When we have a doctor ready to finish his training, he has almost no training in the *human* part of human sexuality. He can tell you how damage to the endothelium (the lining of the blood vessels) can interfere with a man's ability to get an erection, but he can't tell you the first thing about what that performance problem will do to the man's confidence, self-esteem, or sense of masculinity. The problem is that if he doesn't know the questions to ask, or doesn't care about asking them, the doctor will never understand the patient's real problem and therefore never solve the real issue. He will prescribe drugs that treat symptoms but might even make the sexual problems worse!

The human body is composed of numerous systems that all need to work together. It is composed of trillions of miraculous cells, each with its own specialty and function. Those cells need to work together precisely, so they communicate with each other continuously. Can you imagine how complex this task is? But for eighty years and more, it works. The medical profession might understand some of this, but it cannot figure out how to build a single living cell. It is time that we acknowledge that the human being doesn't live inside the cell; it's the living, thinking, feeling person standing in front of us. *That* is who we should be treating.

I would like to see the way medical schools approach sexuality change and adapt to the times we live in. Teach students the anatomical and physiological basis for arousal and orgasm, but also teach them about the emotional, psychological, and social aspects of sexuality. Teach them about the impact of sex on immunity, sleep, and pain. Teach them to respect the importance of happiness and closeness for a person's overall well-being—something most medical schools have no interest in today.

Have students shadow a sex therapist and talk to his or her clients so they can become more comfortable talking with patients about their own sexual issues without embarrassment. Doing these things would make a big difference in how young doctors view sexuality and address it with patients. The goal should be to get young physicians addressing sexuality as comfortably as they take a medical history or take blood pressure.

THE BROKEN SYSTEM

THE OTHER HUGE BARRIER TO physicians spending more time talking with patients about sex is the fact that they don't have very much time to spend with their patients. Young doctors, burdened with high medical school debt, are locked into a system that is against spending time with patients. We are told that efficiency, not quality care, should be our priority. Medicare tell us to place the right code on every diagnosis and service. We are told by the malpractice insurance companies to document everything in electronic medical records as a priority for defense in court. Lawyers tell us how to practice *defensive medicine* so we are protected against malpractice suits. Health insurance companies encourage us to do the opposite—to offer the cheapest treatment possible instead of preventive medicine.

That is what physicians in our country confront every day. Offering real care and personal attention to patients in need—really healing people—is an *afterthought*. It is nearly impossible for young physicians to spend enough time with a patient to deal with something as delicate and personal as sexual problems. In this society, that is a luxury, not a priority. Consequently, sexual problems, as important as they might be, are ignored and overlooked. Patients continue to suffer alone and in silence.

That is why years ago I decided that I would not accept health insurance in most cases. Insurers demand that physicians spend as little time with each patient as they can—just enough time to enter the relevant data and make a quick presumed diagnosis. But I can conduct my examination and ask pertinent questions that will enable me to spot hidden health problems, all while still having time to ask, "So, how is your sex life?" If the patient is male and he says, "We are happy. We have sex two or three times a week, we both reach orgasm, we're very happy and compatible, and I love my wife," then that's the end of it.

But if there is a problem—if I see that telltale pain or shame in the patient's face—then I need to be free to take a lot more time talking with that patient. As I have said, most of the time, the sexual symptoms that the patient is experiencing are the result of emotional stress on the body, and of shame, anger, and frustration. When we talk, when he or she is able to open up about this subject, a weight is lifted. The change in demeanor is always striking, and a change in health and happiness usually follows.

But that is only possible because my patients trust me. I have earned that trust by demonstrating my intention to take care of them by looking at all avenues, including taking the time to ask about their intimate life as well as their other medical problems.

This takes us from physician and patient and turns us into partners, which makes the patient more likely to be open, to listen to my recommendations, and to follow instructions. It doesn't really take much extra time to achieve this and actually saves time later that I would have to use for repetition and unnecessary persuasion.

The average physician will never ask those questions about sexuality, so there will always be an aspect of the patient's health they know nothing about. Most won't even ask about physiological phenomena like ED. They are not rewarded for digging deeper. They either have no interest in the subject, or they simply aren't comfortable with it. In one survey of PCPs, only 4 percent of consultations dealt with sexual concerns.[1]

I was curious, so one day I asked several physicians in my community whether the topic of sexuality ever came up between them and their patients. They all looked at me as if I had dropped in from the moon. They were astonished by my question and said that was a matter for the patient's gynecologist or urologist. But in secret, some of them asked me for Viagra samples, as they were too embarrassed to write a prescription for themselves and possibly didn't want anybody to know . . . even their wives. This is the taboo we're dealing with!

Another problem is the way that medical practices and offices are designed. In the United States, medicine is impersonal and often delivered by machine. Everything is voice mail, mobile apps, and computers. In my day, we found our physicians by asking for referrals from trusted family or friends; now we find them through online reviews. And it is becoming worse, giving the false impression that this body machine is just mechanical without flesh and soul. Sadly, the doctors are delivering their services based on this model.

When patients come to an office for an appointment, they often see physician assistants or nurse practitioners instead of the physician whose name is on the practice. Now, there is nothing wrong with these skilled people, and they are knowledgeable and helpful, but they lack the physician's training, and because they are employees, they may not have the same commitment to the well-being of each patient that a good physician should possess. Moreover, they can never gain the same patient trust as a trained and experienced physician. That is why I take each patient history myself, with no one else in the room. I want the experience for my patients to be more personal, not less. This may take me more time, but I always gain more valuable information about the patient that I could not gain by reviewing notes.

Another way primary care medicine is being made less personal is through technology. Mobile apps like Doctor on Demand and First Opinion let people talk to a licensed physician through their smart phones and ask all sorts of questions about symptoms and possible problems. Now, I'm sure these kinds of solutions are very helpful to people who live in remote areas or small towns where doctors and hospitals are not available for economic reasons, but they are *not* a substitute for sitting down in person with a physician who gets to know you and who you can learn to trust over time.

Today it seems like there is no time for the patient, no respect for the relationship that builds trust and leads to healing by way of the mind. When we do see the doctor, the main concerns of the physicians and office staff seem to be these:

- Avoiding legal liability. Every time a patient comes in with a headache, the physician has to rule out an aneurysm or brain cancer for legal reasons. That's a big reason that

American physicians on the whole order too many tests that waste billions of dollars.[2] We have turned medicine into a mechanical system. For every disorder, there are written instruction on what the physician is supposed to do. We have eliminated the skill, talent, intuition, and art of medicine, making it empty and heartless.

- Creating accurate electronic medical records and doing billing and coding the right way so the doctor will be properly paid by Medicare or the insurance company. Billing alone has become so complex that some medical practices have to hire outside companies to handle it.

None of these things is unimportant. Accurate medical records are crucial to tracking a patient's care over time and preventing errors. No doctor wants to be sued. And obviously, every physician should be fairly compensated for his or her work. However, all these things should be secondary to the practice of good medicine, and too often they have become more important. The patient is an afterthought—almost an annoyance. No wonder physicians don't take the time to talk about sexuality; they barely have the time to talk about anything! It is not surprising that more than 50 percent of all physicians in this country plan to retire within the next few years, and more than 60 percent say they suffer from burnout.

WHAT NEEDS TO CHANGE?

HEALTH CARE SHOULD BE A PARTNERSHIP between patient and physician. You should work together, teaching each other about what works for you—not just in your sex life but in your entire life. The physician is the skilled advisor with the years of training, making recommendations based on science and experience. The patient is actually doing the work: making the lifestyle changes, doing the exercise, being more intimate with his or her partner. Together, physician and patient should learn how to help the patient live long and well. That's impossible with a system that rewards brief, impersonal encounters—medical *transactions*, really.

Take sexually transmitted disease. There are about 20 million cases each year in the United States, and most of those happen because of a lack of knowledge among women and men about how to prevent it. Take a subject that is already taboo—sex—and create a system where doctors and patients are discouraged from talking about anything more than the superficial. Nobody ever gets comfortable talking about sensitive subjects. As a result, you might have a doctor ready to finish his training who knows nothing about sexuality or how to talk about it. I don't blame these doctors because when you don't do something for a long time, you don't know how to do it. But I do blame medical educators. To turn out physicians who are so unprepared to talk about an experience that is so central to human well-being is inexcusable.

Health care in the United States is also being run by lawyers. Everything now is about avoiding liability. If a patient comes in with a headache, you have to send him for an MRI or CT scan before even having a discussion. The liability insurance companies literally say, "If you don't do this, we'll not cover you for a lawsuit."

There's an incentive to spend money and a disincentive to listen to the patient and use common sense and experience to figure out what the problem might be. We've created a monster, a restrictive system in which a doctor who doesn't see five patients an hour will not be able to keep his doors open.

The solution is not to reform the existing system. The only real solution is to let the existing system collapse and then to replace that system with a single-payer, government-run system. These function well in many countries, including Israel, and this type of system is probably the best for changing how physicians and patients interact. Because the physician is paid by a single source, and no insurance companies are involved, he or she does not have that incentive to see five patients each hour. The physician can slow down, engage with the patient, and yes, talk about sexuality. He or she can actually practice medicine, which is what we got into the profession to do.

Socialized medicine is not perfect. Some patients might have to wait a few months for certain procedures. But they will get care at low or no additional cost, and people with wealth will still be able to go to their private doctor and inject a great deal of capital into the health system. That will subsidize the care for everybody else. Many of those people are the ones who come to my practice. I don't accept many types of insurance, and they pay me out of pocket. This gives me the freedom to focus all my time and attention on them so I can get to know them and ask things like, "How is your sex life with your spouse?" As I have made clear, that is a question that can change people's lives.

Change begins on both the patient side and the physician side. Patients need to be proactive and bring their complaints about time and physician engagement to the attention of their doctors and insurers. They need to insist on more time to talk about issues like their sexuality, and if their physician cannot or will not do this, they need to be prepared to move on to someone else.

Physicians need to find a way to spend an extra few minutes to learn more about each patient's sexual life and possible sexual disorders. This might seem to go against the practical need for the physician to make a living, but it really does not. For example, by helping my patients address their sexual issues with communication and greater intimacy, I have helped thousands of them to stop taking medications for depression, anxiety, and the like. That creates real cost savings for insurers, makes patients happy, and saves doctors' time. This really does work!

HOW DO WE CHANGE IT?

I DON'T THINK WAITING FOR the system to fail and for socialized medicine to take over is the only way to change things. Patients can bring about change by demanding it, and medical schools can change how future doctors view sexuality by changing how they teach. They can start shaping young students' view that sex is a positive, essential part of life, an organic aspect of the human mental and physiological system, and a gift. As such, we have to respect it, know about it, and learn what it can do for us. Schools should train students in the impact of sexuality on mood, stress hormones, depression, anxiety, metabolism, sleep, self-image, and much more. Sex is not a side effect of our biology; it is a powerful determining factor in how we live.

Schools need to break the taboo about these topics. There should be no taboo topics in medical schools as long as there is science to back up the teachings! If the taboo is broken for young physicians, they will help their patients break the taboo in turn by talking about sexuality in their appointments. That will help patients see the logic in getting help. If you have a stomach problem, you go to your gastroenterologist; if you have a heart problem, you see your cardiologist. If you have a sex problem, you see your PCP.

I would like to see people bringing their sexual questions and concerns to their physicians become as commonplace as people going to the doctor for their acid reflux or high blood pressure. That starts with the physicians. Even older ones long out of medical school can change how they do things. The more they talk about sexuality, the more they will do research, and the more they will learn. At the end of the day, all physicians want to help their patients.

Following the path of sexuality to the root cause of symptoms like palpitations, skin rashes, insomnia, muscle pain, and anxiety will also allow doctors to find solutions and effective treatments much faster. I cannot tell you how many times I spoke to men and women who went to doctor after doctor for years trying to find the cause of their fatigue or depression. They spent countless hours and lots of money, experimented with prescriptions, and tried many things that did not work.

The reason was obvious: the root cause was the stress and emotional pain caused by their sexual dysfunction and the damage to their marriage—but no one ever asked them about that. Focusing on sexuality enabled me to help people find relief a lot faster and a lot easier. Patients are eager to participate in this, but they are afraid to initiate the conversation, and the physician is not asking the right questions.

I had one patient who was running from one physician to another with multiple somatic symptoms, afraid that every one of them was associated with major disease. This forty-two-year-old man, good looking and healthy, was single and had no sexual activity. I noticed that he had lost his self-confidence, was swarmed by fear and anxiety, and had problems sleeping, which is unusual in a young man. When I got to my sexuality questions, he became angry and declined to speak about it, but then admitted that he had no sexual activity because he was ashamed of his genitalia. After cooling off, he let me examine him, and I found nothing wrong with his genitalia.

When I told him that he was fine, he calmed down and told me his story. Apparently, as a boy at summer camp, other boys laughed at him for having a small penis. Since that moment, he had never exposed his genitalia because he believed he was abnormal. He also turned his fear and shame into the physical symptoms that led him to so many doctors and tests.

No physician ever asked him about his sexuality or attempted to examine him. He told me that he envied other young people who got married and had kids but felt sorry for himself that his bad luck deprived him of this part of life. Isn't that heartbreaking? When I told him that his penis was totally normal, he broke into tears of relief and happiness. It took several more meetings, but eventually his somatic symptoms faded away, he gained confidence, and was able to sleep well. Six months later, he shared with me a photo of his girlfriend, and one year later he proudly showed me his beautiful four-month-old baby girl.

That is a good outcome, but why did this young man have to suffer for so long? He was a victim of sexual secrecy, of a medical system that excludes the sexual system from its questions, examinations, and tests. It is hard to believe that this is happening in our new world of freedom of expression, sexual liberation, and advanced medical science, but it is.

It is important that we bring back human touch to medicine. Of course, the physician will touch the patient when doing a physical exam, but I am talking about touch that is comforting and human. In this era when so many people are being accused of sexual harassment, many physicians are terrified to touch their patients for fear of being sued. They create distance from their patients as a way of practicing. I heard this repeatedly from patients, who complained that their other doctors did not look at them, listen to them, examine them, or even touch them. They just took a medical history, wrote a prescription, and left the room.

That is not medicine. You cannot practice medicine effectively without touching your patients. You will be unable to diagnose him, and you will demonstrate no compassion and earn no trust. Touch can help connect me to a patient and create trust, and I have achieved that with many of my patients. Women tend to need it more. They come in with pain and a lot of anxiety, and if I put my arm around their shoulder, they know it's not sexual. I am trying to bring them comfort, to say with touch, "I am here for you. I care about you, and together we are going to find a solution to what troubles you." Touch by itself is healing.

Once the physician finds the courage to talk with his patients about sexual issues, he will be fascinated by how much emotion comes out, how much suffering is involved, and how much helpful information will be revealed to him. When he knows this aspect of his patients, he will be able to develop more trusting relationships with them, which will lead to better diagnoses and real healing.

I never walk into a room with a patient, male or female, without either shaking hands or putting my arm on their shoulders. I have never once felt that it made the patient uncomfortable. On the contrary, patients come to expect the gesture, in particular the women because it comforts them to feel I am on their side. It lets them know that our time is not about lawyers and insurance companies or about me trying to protect myself. It is about them, about me learning about them and helping them find healing.

What else can physicians do?

- Physicians and educators can maintain an open mind and acknowledge that an understanding of the whole person— not just the physiological systems—is necessary to help people achieve true wellness, health, vitality, and happiness. This is how we can become genuine healers rather than people who write prescriptions and order tests.

- We must find new ways to compensate physicians so they are not compensated just by the number of patients they see per hour but also based on their experience and effectiveness at keeping people healthy over the long term and preventing chronic disease.

- We also need to change the system to ensure that all Americans have health coverage and can afford to see a doctor to talk about anything that bothers them, including sexual dysfunction. The United States spends more per capita on health care than any other nation but has poorer outcomes than most, and even with the Affordable Care Act, in 2019 there were still more than twenty-eight million Americans with no health insurance. That must change in order for people to have access to care and advice about their sex lives.

- Begin to change how medical schools teach students about sexuality. We should be teaching that sex is an essential part of the overall picture of good health and important to well-being and a positive psychology. Medical professionals must be taught to respect sex, not to snicker at it.

- We need to get more good information to the public and encourage people to talk to their doctors about their sex lives. That can begin with better sex education, but it needs to continue through books like this one, newspapers and magazines, TV shows, and the Internet. Insurance companies should communicate with their customers and suggest that they talk to their doctors about their ED and orgasms as easily as they talk about their cholesterol and arthritis.

- Patients and physicians should demand that insurers pay for counseling for sexual disorders and for sex therapy as easily as they pay for physical therapy.

- We could also create incentives for physicians to talk about sexuality, maybe by creating new specialties focused on sexuality. Imagine older patients going to sex specialists just for help with their sex lives. Access to this type of physician would improve the health and happiness of everyone.

But let's start small. Physicians, spend five minutes more with each patient and ask them about their sex lives and their relationships. Start today. You will build trust, get to know your patients better, help more people, enjoy your work more, and be better doctors. Patients, insist on spending a few minutes talking with your doctor about your sex life at your next physical. Don't accept the "fifteen minutes and a nurse practitioner" approach to medicine. You're the patient. This is all supposed to be for you. If you demand better, it will happen.

Change is possible. I know because I have seen it. But it will take creativity, hard work, openness to change, humility on the part of physicians, and persistence on the part of patients. But it can happen. Together, we can help millions of people enjoy better sex and better lives.

ENDNOTES

INTRODUCTION

1   Sy Mukherjee, "Viagra Just Turned 20. Here's How Much Money the ED Drug Makes," *Fortune*, March 27, 2018.

2   Milton Lakin and Hadley Wood, "Erectile Dysfunction," Cleveland Clinic Center for Continuing Education, June 2018.

3   Debby Herbenick et al., "Women's Experiences With Genital Touching, Sexual Pleasure, and Orgasm: Results From a U.S. Probability Sample of Women Ages 18 to 94," *Journal of Sex & Marital Therapy* 44, no. 2 (2018) 201–212.

4   D. L. Rowland, L. M. Cempel, and A. R. Tempel, "Women's Attributions Regarding Why They Have Difficulty Reaching Orgasm," *Journal of Sex & Marital Therapy* 44, no. 5 (2018): 475–484.

5   Edward O. Laumann et al. "A cross-national study of subjective sexual well-being among older women and men: findings from the Global Study of Sexual Attitudes and Behaviors," *Archives of Sexual Behavior* 35, no. 2 (April 2006): 145–161. Published online April 26 2006.

6   "Sexual Dysfunction and Disease," Cleveland Clinic, my.clevelandclinic. org/health/diseases/9125-sexual-dysfunction-and-disease, retrieved May 29, 2019.

CHAPTER ONE: WHY DON'T WE TALK ABOUT SEX?

1   Jean M. Twenge, Ryne A. Sherman, and Brooke E. Wells, "Declines in Sexual Frequency among American Adults, 1989–2014," *Archives of Sexual Behavior*, (2017) 46. 10.1007/s10508-017-0953-1.

2   Kate Julian, "Why Are Young People Having So Little Sex?" *The Atlantic*, December 2018, www.theatlantic.com/magazine/archive/2018/12/the-sex-recession/573949/, retrieved May 30, 2019.

3   "Marriage and Divorce," American Psychological Association, www.apa. org/topics/divorce, retrieved May 30, 2019.

4   US Bureau of Labor Statistics, "Employment in families with children in 2016," April 27, 2017, www.bls.gov/opub/ted/2017/employment-in-families-with-children-in-2016.htm, retrieved May 30, 2019.

5   William A. Fisher et al., "Individual and Partner Correlates of Sexual Satisfaction and Relationship Happiness in Midlife Couples: Dyadic Analysis of the International Survey of Relationships," *Archives of Sexual Behavior* 44, no. 6, (August 2015): 1609–1620. Published online November 5, 2014.

6   Audun Vik and Mette Brekke, "Do patients consult their GP for sexual concerns? A cross sectional explorative study." *Scandinavian Journal of Primary Health Care* 35, no. 4 (December 2017): 373–378.

7   Evan Atlantis and Thomas Sullivan, "Bidirectional association between depression and sexual dysfunction: a systematic review and meta-analysis," *Journal of Sexual Medicine* 9, no.6 (June 2012): 1497–1507. Published online March 29, 2012.

8   Kara Mayer Robinson, "10 Surprising Health Benefits of Sex," WebMD, www.webmd.com/sex-relationships/guide/sex-and-health#1, retrieved May 30, 2019.

9   Gerard F. Anderson, Peter Hussey, and Varduhi Petrosyan, "It's Still the Prices, Stupid: Why the US Spends So Much on Health Care, and a Tribute to Uwe Reinhardt," *Health Affairs* 38, no. 1 (January 2019).

10 Janice Zarro Brodman, *Sex Rules!: Astonishing Sexual Practices and Gender Roles Around the World*, (Coral Gables, FL: Mango, 2017).

11 "The Effects of Stress on Your Body," WedMD, December 10, 2017, www.webmd.com/balance/stress-management/effects-of-stress-on-your-body, retrieved June 3, 2019.

12 "New National Sexual Health Survey Reveals Barriers to Addressing Issues," American Sexual Health Association, http://www.ashasexualhealth.org/new-national-sexual-health-survey, retrieved June 3, 2019.

13 Julian, "Why Are Young People Having So Little Sex?"

14 Anik Debrot et al., "More Than Just Sex: Affection Mediates the Association Between Sexual Activity and Well-Being," *Personality and Social Psychology Bulletin* 43, no. 3 (March 2017): 287–299.

15 Adena M. Galinsky and Linda J. Waite, "Sexual Activity and Psychological Health as Mediators of the Relationship Between Physical Health and Marital quality," *The Journals of Gerontology Series B: Psychological Sciences and Social Sciences* 69, no.3 (2014): 482–92.

16 "National Poll on Healthy Aging," University of Michigan Institute for Healthcare Policy and Innovation, May 2018, deepblue.lib.umich.edu/bitstream/handle/2027.42/143212/NPHA-Sexual-Health-Report_050118_final.pdf, retrieved June 3, 2019.

17 Amy Muise, Ulrich Schimmack, and Emily A. Impett, Sexual Frequency Predicts Greater Well-Being, But More Is Not Always Better. *Social Psychological and Personality Science* 7, no. 4 (November 2015).

18 "Sex Is the Biggest Cause of Divorce," Woolley & Co Solicitors, September 2, 2008, www.bedfordtoday.co.uk/news/sex-is-biggest-cause-of-divorce-1-1094645, retrieved June 3, 2019

19 Susan A. Hall et al., "Sexual Activity, Erectile Dysfunction, and Incident Cardiovascular Events," *American Journal of Cardiology* 105, no. 2 (January 2015): 192–197.

20 Zhiming Cheng and Russell Smyth, "Sex and happiness," *Journal of Economic Behavior & Organization* 112 (April 2015): 26–32.

21 Michelle Overman, "Can Sexual Frustration Lead to Depression?" eCoun-seling.com, February 14, 2019, www.e-counseling.com/depression/sexu-al-frustration-and-depression, retrieved June 3, 2019.

CHAPTER TWO: FORTY-FIVE YEARS OF TREATING A SILENT EPIDEMIC

1   R. Butler et al., "Estimating Time Physicians and Other Health Care Workers Spend with Patients in an Intensive Care Unit Using a Sensor Network," *The American Journal of Medicine* 131, no. 8 (August 2011):972. e9–972.e15. doi: 10.1016/j.amjmed.2018.03.015. Epub 2018 Apr 9.

2   Rekha Mankad, "Coronary artery spasm: Cause for concern?" Mayo Clinic, January 9, 2019, www.mayoclinic.org/diseases-conditions/angina/ expert-answers/coronary-artery-spasm/faq-20058316, retrieved June 5, 2019.

3   John Mulhall et al., "Importance of and Satisfaction with Sex Among Men and Women Worldwide: Results of the Global Better Sex Survey," *The Journal of Sexual Medicine* 5, no. 4 (April 2008): 788–795.

4   "50 Common Signs and Symptoms of Stress," The American Institute of Stress, www.stress.org/stress-effects, retrieved June 5, 2019.

5   S. Chetty et. al., "Stress and glucocorticoids promote oligodendrogenesis in the adult hippocampus," *Molecular Psychiatry* 19, no. 12 (December 2014): 1275–1283.

6   J. F. Sheridan et al., "Psychoneuroimmunology: stress effects on pathogen-esis and immunity during infection." *Clinical Microbiology Reviews* 7, no. 2 (1994): 200–212.

7   Paul E. Marik and Rinaldo Bellomo, "Stress hyperglycemia: an essential survival response!." *Critical care (London, England)* 17, no. 2 (March 2013): 305. doi:10.1186/cc12514.

8   Jo Marchant, "Placebos: Honest fakery," *Nature* 535 (July 14, 2016): S14–15.

9   Pauline Anderson, "Doctors' Suicide Rate Highest of Any Profession," WebMD, May 8, 2018, www.webmd.com/mental-health/news/20180508/ doctors-suicide-rate-highest-of-any-profession#1, retrieved June 5, 2019.

10 Jean Decety and Aikaterini Fotopoulou, "Why empathy has a beneficial impact on others in medicine: unifying theories," *Frontiers in Behavioral Neuroscience* 8 (January 14, 2015): 457.

CHAPTER THREE: TWO DIFFERENT MACHINES

1 Elisabeth A. Lloyd, *The Case of the Female Orgasm: Bias in the Science of Evolution*, (Cambridge: Harvard University Press, 2005).

2 Debby Herbenick et al., "Women's Experiences with Genital Touching, Sexual Pleasure, and Orgasm: Results from a U.S. Probability Sample of Women Ages 18 to 94", *Journal of Sex & Marital Therapy* 44, no. 2 (February 17, 2018): 201–212.

3 Lauren Mazzo, "The Best Way to Work Out to Increase Your Sex Drive," *Shape,* March 11, 2019, www.shape.com/lifestyle/sex-and-love/best-work-out-increase-sex-drive, retrieved June 12, 2019.

4 Ross Pomeroy, "What Penis Size Do Women Prefer?" Real Clear Science, September 7, 2015, www.realclearscience.com/journal_club/2015/09/08/what_penis_size_do_women_prefer_109375.html, retrieved June 12, 2019.

5 Herbenick, "Women's Experiences with Genital Touching, Sexual Pleasure, and Orgasm."

6 Osmo Kontula and Anneli Miettinen, "Determinants of female sexual orgasms," *Socioaffective Neuroscience & Psychology* 6 (October 2016).

CHAPTER FOUR: MEN AND ERECTILE DYSFUNCTION: A CRISIS OF SECRECY

1 Cecilia Tasca et al. "Women and Hysteria in the History of Mental Health." *Clinical Practice and Epidemiology in Mental Health* 8 (2012):110–119.

2 Domenico Santoro et al., "Impotence in the 18th and 19th century: concepts of etiology and approaches to therapy," Journal of Nephrology 22 Suppl. 14 (Nov–Dec 2009): 67–70.

3 Suzanne K. Chambers et al, "Erectile dysfunction, masculinity, and psychosocial outcomes: a review of the experiences of men after prostate cancer treatment." *Translational Andrology and Urology* 6, no. 1 (2017): 60–68.

4   Giulia Rastrelli and Mario Maggi, "Erectile dysfunction in fit and healthy young men: psychological or pathological?." *Translational Andrology and Urology* 6, no. 1 (2017): 79–90. doi:10.21037/tau.2016.09.06

5   Patrick J. Skerrett, "Erectile dysfunction often a warning sign of heart disease," Harvard Medical School: Harvard Health Publishing, www. health.harvard.edu/blog/erectile-dysfunction-often-a-warning-sign-of-heart-disease-201110243648, October 24, 2011, retrieved June 14, 2019.

6   Dennis Thompson, "Study Sees Link Between Porn and Sexual Dysfunction," WebMD, May 12, 2017, www.webmd.com/sex/news/20170512/study-sees-link-between-porn-and-sexual-dysfunction#1, retrieved June 14, 2019.

7   "Benefits of exercise for the prostate and erectile dysfunction help," Harvard Medical School: Harvard Health Publishing, May 2007, https://www.health.harvard.edu/press_releases/benefits-of-exercise-for-the-prostate

8   H. A. Feldman et al., "Impotence and its medical and psychosocial correlates: results of the Massachusetts Male Aging Study," *The Journal of Urology* 151, no. 1 (January 1994): 54–61.

9   Rastrelli, "Erectile dysfunction in fit and healthy young men: psychological or pathological?"

10 J. R. Kovac et al., "Effects of cigarette smoking on erectile dysfunction." *Andrologia* 47, no. 10 (2015): 1087–92.

11 "Dietary supplements for erectile dysfunction: A natural treatment for ED?" Mayo Clinic, January 26, 2019, www.mayoclinic.org/diseases-conditions/erectile-dysfunction/in-depth/erectile-dysfunction-herbs/art-20044394, retrieved June 14, 2019.

12 Elodie J. O'Connor et al., "Attitudes and Experiences: Qualitative Perspectives on Erectile Dysfunction from the Female Partner," *Journal of Health Psychology* 17, no. 1 (January 2012): 3–13.

13 Barbara Chubak, Barbara, "Impotence and Suing for Sex in Eighteenth-Century England," *Urology* 71, no. 3, (March 2008): 480–484.

14 William A. Fisher et al., "Sexual experience of female partners of men with erectile dysfunction: the female experience of men's attitudes to life events and sexuality (FEMALES) study." *Journal of Sexual Medicine* 2, no. 5 (September 2005): 675–684.

15 Hongjun Li, Tiejun Gao, Run Wang, "The role of the sexual partner in managing erectile dysfunction," *Nature Reviews Urology* 13, no. 3 (March 2016): 168–177. Published online Feb. 2, 2016.

CHAPTER FIVE: WHY WOMEN SHOULD TREAT SEX LIKE GOING TO THE GYM

1 Dana R. Ambler, E. J. Bieber, and M. P. Diamond, "Sexual function in elderly women: a review of current literature." *Reviews in Obstetrics and Gynecology* 5, no. 1 (2012): 16–27.

2 Cindy Günzler and Michael M. Berner, "Efficacy of psychosocial interventions in men and women with sexual dysfunctions—a systematic review of controlled clinical trials: part 2—the efficacy of psychosocial interventions for female sexual dysfunction," *Journal of Sexual Medicine* 9, no. 12 (December 2012): 3108–3125. Published online Oct. 22, 2012.

3 I. Goldstein et al., "Hypoactive Sexual Desire Disorder: International Society for the Study of Women's Sexual Health (ISSWSH) Expert Consensus Panel Review," *Mayo Clinical Proceedings* 92, no. 1 (January 2017):114–128. doi: 10.1016/j.mayocp.2016.09.018. Epub 2016 Dec 1.

4 Debby Herbenick et al., "Sexual diversity in the United States: Results from a nationally representative probability sample of adult women and men," PLOS ONE 12, no.7 (July 20, 2017): e0181198. https://doi.org/10.1371/journal.pone.0181198.

5 Rosemary Basson, "Sexual Desire and Arousal Disorders in Women," April 6, 2006, *New England Journal of Medicine* 354:1497–1506.

6 Jan L. Shifren, et al., "Sexual Problems and Distress in United States Women: Prevalence and Correlates," *Obstetrics & Gynecology*, 112, no. 5 (November 2008): 970–978.

7 Basson, "Sexual Desire and Arousal Disorders in Women."

8 R. L. Smith, L. Gallicchio, and J. A. Flaws, "Factors Affecting Sexual Function in Midlife Women: Results from the Midlife Women's Health Study," *Journal of Women's Health (Larchmt)*, 26, no. 9 (September 2017): 923–932. doi: 10.1089/jwh.2016.6135. Epub Feb. 28, 2017.

9 R. T. Segraves et al., "Bupropion sustained release (SR) for the treatment of hypoactive sexual desire disorder (HSDD) in nondepressed women," *Journal of Sex and Marital Therapy* 27, no. 3 (May 2001): 303–16.

10 Rashmi Baid, and Rakesh Agarwal, "Flibanserin: A controversial drug for female hypoactive sexual desire disorder," *Industrial Psychiatry Journal* 27, no. 1 (2018): 154–157. doi:10.4103/ipj.ipj_20_16.

11 Cindy Günzler and Michael M. Berner, "Efficacy of psychosocial interventions in men and women with sexual dysfunctions—a systematic review of controlled clinical trials: part 2—the efficacy of psychosocial interventions for female sexual dysfunction," *Journal of Sexual Medicine* 9, no. 12 (2012): 3108–3125.

12 Lia M. Jiannine, "An investigation of the relationship between physical fitness, self-concept, and sexual functioning," *Journal of Education and Health Promotion* 7, no. 57 (May 3, 2018).

13 Vikas Dhikav et al., "Yoga in Female Sexual Functions," *The Journal of Sexual Medicine* 7, no. 2, pt. 2, (2010): 964–970.

14 Mas Sahidayana Mohktar et al., "A quantitative approach to measure women's sexual function using electromyography: a preliminary study of the Kegel exercise." *Medical Science Monitor* 19 (December 13, 2013): 1159–66.

15 Lisa Dawn Hamilton, and Cindy M. Meston, "Chronic stress and sexual function in women, *The Journal of Sexual Medicine* 10, 10 (2013): 2443–54. doi:10.1111/jsm.12249.

CHAPTER SIX: COMMUNICATION IS THE KEY

1 Noam Shpancer, "Why Aren't We Talking to Our Partners About Sex?" *Psychology Today*, March 31, 2014, www.psychologytoday.com/us/blog/insight-therapy/201403/why-arent-we-talking-our-partners-about-sex, retrieved June 23, 2019.

2 Susan Heitler, "What Does Communication Have to Do with a Good Relationship?" Good Therapy, June 3, 2010, www.goodtherapy.org/blog/what-does-communication-have-to-do-with-good-relationship, retrieved June 23, 2019.

3 Jennifer L. Montesi et al., "The Specific Importance of Communicating about Sex to Couples' Sexual and Overall Relationship Satisfaction." *Journal of Social and Personal Relationships* 28, no. 5 (August 2011): 591–609.

4   Harriet Lerner, "Should You Have Sex With Your Spouse When You Don't Want To?" *Psychology Today*, January 27, 2019, www.psychologytoday.com/us/blog/the-dance-connection/201901/should-you-have-sex-your-spouse-when-you-dont-want, retrieved June 24, 2019.

5   Sabna Kotta, Shahid H. Ansari, and Javed Ali, "Exploring scientifically proven herbal aphrodisiacs," *Pharmacognosy Review* 7, no. 13 (2013): 1–10. doi:10.4103/0973-7847.112832.

CHAPTER SEVEN: SEXUAL HEALTH EQUALS TOTAL WELL-BEING

1   "CDC/HRSA Advisory Committee on HIV, Viral Hepatitis, and STD Prevention and Treatment," Centers for Disease Control and Prevention, https://www.cdc.gov/maso/facm/facmCHACHSPT.html.

2   Carl J. Charnetski and Francis X. Brennan, "Sexual frequency and salivary immunoglobulin A (IgA)," *Psychology Report* 94, no. 3, pt. 1 (June 2004): 839–844.

3   Anke Hambach et al., "The Impact of Sexual Activity on Idiopathic Headaches: An Observational Study." *Cephalalgia* 33, no. 6 (April 2013): 384–389.

4   Susan A. Hall et al., "Sexual Activity, Erectile Dysfunction, and Incident Cardiovascular Events," *American Journal of Cardiology* 105, no. 2 (January 15, 2010): 192–197.

5   "Ejaculation frequency and prostate cancer," Harvard Medical School: Harvard Health Publishing, March 2014, updated June 19, 2019, www.health.harvard.edu/mens-health/ejaculation_frequency_and_prostate_cancer, retrieved June 24, 2019.

6   Michele Lastella et al., "Sex and Sleep: Perceptions of Sex as a Sleep Promoting Behavior in the General Adult Population," *Frontiers in Public Health* 7, no. 33 (2019).

7   Jose Devasia and Neha Dasgupta, "Protests Erupt in India After Women Defy Menstruation Ban at Hindu Temple," HuffPost, January 2, 2019, www.huffpost.com/entry/protests-erupt-in-india-after-women-defy-menstruation-ban-at-hindu-temple_n_5c2cbeb8e4b0407e9086baef, retrieved June 24, 2019.

8   Heather Hensman Kettrey, "'How can women feel comfortable saying no when they are told they can't say yes?" The Conversation, February 16, 2018, https://theconversation.com/how-can-women-feel-comfortable-saying-no-when-they-are-told-they-cant-say-yes-91613.

9   Nick Drydakis, "The effect of sexual activity on wages," *International Journal of Manpower*, 36, no. 2 (May 2015): 192–215.

CHAPTER EIGHT: BETTER SEX AS WE AGE? YES!

1   Emmanuele A. Jannini and Rossella E. Nappi, "Couplepause: A New Paradigm in Treating Sexual Dysfunction During Menopause and Andropause," *Sexual Medicine Reviews* 6, no. 3 (2018): 384–395.

2   Preeti Malani and Erica Solway, "National Poll on Healthy Aging," University of Michigan, May 3, 2018, www.healthyagingpoll.org/report/lets-talk-about-sex, retrieved June 25, 2019.

3   William R. Rowley et al., "Diabetes 2030: Insights from Yesterday, Today, and Future Trends," *Population Health Management* 20, no. 1 (2017): 6–12; doi:10.1089/pop.2015.0181.

4   Ihab, Younis et al., "Can obesity affect female sexuality?" *Human Andrology* 3, no. 4 (December 2013): 98–106.

5   B. J. Chandler and S. Brown, "Sex and relationship dysfunction in neurological disability," *Journal of Neurology, Neurosurgery & Psychiatry* 65, no. 6 (1998): 877–880.

6   B. Plassman et al., "Prevalence of Dementia in the United States: The Aging, Demographics, and Memory Study," *Neuroepidemiology* 29, no. 1–2 (November 2007): 125–132.

7   Yanping Li, et. al., "Impact of Healthy Lifestyle Factors on Life Expectancies in the US Population," *Circulation* 138, no. 4 (April 2018); 345–355, https://doi.org/10.1161/CIRCULATIONAHA.117.032047.

8   Diane Lange, "Challenges to Intimacy: Iris Krasnow On Sex After 60, 70, 80," Senior Planet, March 3, 2014, seniorplanet.org/challenges-to-intimacy-iris-krasnow-on-sex-after-60-70-and-80, retrieved June 26, 2019.

9   Lee Smith et al., "Sexual Activity Is Associated with Greater Enjoyment of Life in Older Adults," *Sexual Medicine* 7, no. 1 (2019): 11–18.

CHAPTER NINE: TIME TO BREAK THE TABOO

1   Kathrin F. Stanger-Hall, and David W. Hall, "Abstinence-Only Education and Teen Pregnancy Rates: Why We Need Comprehensive Sex Education in the U.S." *PloS One* 6, no. 10 (2011).

2   Kelli Stidham Hall et al., "The State of Sex Education in the United States." *The Journal of Adolescent Health* 58, no. 6 (2016): 595–7.

3   "The Best Intentions: Unintended Pregnancy and the Well-Being of Children and Families, Committee on Unintended Pregnancy, 1995," Institute of Medicine, The National Academies Press.

4   "Fact Sheet: Female Infertility," Office of Population Affairs, U.S. Dept. of Health and Human Services, www.hhs.gov/opa/reproductive-health/fact-sheets/female-infertility/index.html, retrieved June 27, 2019.

5   David Carter, "Comprehensive Sex Education for Teens Is More Effective than Abstinence," *AJN: American Journal of Nursing* 112, no. 3 (March 2012): 15.

6   Chelsea Ritschel, "Abstinence-only sex education increases teen pregnancy in conservative US states, study finds," *Independent*, February 4, 2019, www.independent.co.uk/news/world/americas/abstinence-sex-education-us-teen-pregnancy-rates-states-a8763051.html, retrieved June 27, 2019.

7   "Birth Control Has Expanded Opportunity for Women," Planned Parenthood, June 2015, www.plannedparenthood.org/files/1614/3275/8659/BC_factsheet_may2015_updated_1.pdf.

8   "Sexually transmitted disease? At my age?" Harvard Medical School: Harvard Health Publishing, February 2018, www.health.harvard.edu/diseases-and-conditions/sexually-transmitted-disease-at-my-age, retrieved June 27, 2019.

CHAPTER TEN: THE BASHFUL PHYSICIAN

1   Audun Vik and Mette Brekke, "Do patients consult their GP for sexual concerns? A cross sectional explorative study" *Scandinavian Journal of Primary Heath Care* 35, no. 4: 373-378.

2   "Unnecessary medical tests, treatments cost $200 billion annually, cause harm," Kaiser Health News, *Healthcare Finance*, May 24, 2017, www.healthcarefinancenews.com/news/unnecessary-medical-tests-treatments-cost-200-billion-annually-cause-harm, retrieved June 28, 2019.